# *ESSENTIALS* on GENETICS AND GENOMICS FOR NURSES

**Kimberly A. Subasic, PhD, MS, BSN, CNE,** is a professor and an Endowed Chair for the Swain Department of Nursing at The Citadel, in Charleston, South Carolina. She received her nursing education at Saint Francis University, the University of Massachusetts Worcester, and Saint Louis University. Her interest in genetics began during her master's education and continued as a focus of her doctoral research. As a graduate of the National Institutes of Health Summer Genetics Institute and the National Institutes of Health, Faculty Champions in Genetics and Genomics, she embraces the benefits of genomics in the provision of person-centered healthcare. Dr. Subasic has been a longstanding member of the International Society of Nurses in genetics (ISONG) and has served on various committees. She has multiple publications and presentations related to genomics. Her clinical experience includes trauma, cardiac, medical-surgical, geriatric, community, and rehabilitative nursing.

# OTHER *ESSENTIALS* BOOKS

Essentials on **ADOLESCENT HEALTH FOR NURSING AND HEALTH PROFESSIONALS**: A Care Guide (*Herrman*)

Essentials for the **ADULT-GERONTOLOGY ACUTE CARE NURSE PRACTITIONER** (*Carpenter*)

Essentials for the **ANTEPARTUM AND POSTPARTUM NURSE**: A Nursing Orientation and Care Guide (*Davidson*)

Essentials Workbook for **CARDIAC DYSRHYTHMIAS AND 12-LEAD EKGs** (*Desmarais*)

Essentials for the **CARDIAC SURGERY NURSE**: Caring for Cardiac Surgery Patients, Third Edition (*Hodge*)

Essentials for **CAREER SUCCESS IN NURSING**: Making the Most of Mentoring (*Vance*)

Essentials for the **CATH LAB NURSE**, Second Edition (*McCulloch*)

Essentials for the **CLASSROOM NURSING INSTRUCTOR**: Classroom Teaching (*Yoder-Wise, Kowalski*)

Essentials for the **CLINICAL NURSE LEADER** (*Wilcox, Deerhake*)

Essentials for the **CLINICAL NURSE MANAGER**: Managing a Changing Workplace, Second Edition (*Fry*)

Essentials for the **CLINICAL NURSING INSTRUCTOR**: Clinical Teaching, Third Edition (*Kan, Stabler-Haas*)

Essentials on **COMBATING NURSE BULLYING, INCIVILITY, AND WORKPLACE VIOLENCE**: What Nurses Need to Know (*Ciocco*)

Essentials About **COMPETENCY-BASED EDUCATION IN NURSING**: How to Teach Competency Mastery (*Wittmann-Price, Gittings*)

Essentials for the **CRITICAL CARE NURSE**, Second Edition (*Hewett*)

Essentials About **CURRICULUM DEVELOPMENT IN NURSING**: How to Develop and Evaluate Educational Programs, Second Edition (*McCoy, Anema*)

Essentials for **DEMENTIA CARE**: What Nurses Need to Know, Second Edition (*Miller*)

Essentials for **DEVELOPING A NURSING ACADEMIC PORTFOLIO**: What You Really Need to Know (*Wittmann-Price*)

Essentials About **DIVERSITY, EQUITY, AND INCLUSION IN NURSING**: Building Competencies for an Antiracism Practice (*Davis*)

Essentials for **DNP ROLE DEVELOPMENT**: A Career Navigation Guide (*Menonna-Quinn, Tortorella Genova*)

Essentials About **EKGs FOR NURSES**: The Rules of Identifying EKGs (*Landrum*)

Essentials for the **ER NURSE**: Guide to a Successful Emergency Department Orientation, Fourth Edition (*Buettner*)

Essentials for **EVIDENCE-BASED PRACTICE IN NURSING**: Third Edition (*Godshall*)

Essentials for the **FAITH COMMUNITY NURSE**: Implementing FCN/Parish Nursing (*Hickman*)

Essentials About **FORENSIC NURSING**: What You Need to Know (*Scannell*)

Essentials on **GENETICS AND GENOMICS FOR NURSES**: Practical Applications (*Subasic*)

Essentials for the **GERONTOLOGY NURSE**: A Nursing Care Guide (*Eliopoulos*)

Essentials About **GI AND LIVER DISEASES FOR NURSES**: What APRNs Need to Know (*Chaney*)

Essentials About the **GYNECOLOGICAL EXAM**: A Professional Guide for NPs, PAs, and Midwives, Second Edition (*Secor, Fantasia*)

Essentials in **HEALTH INFORMATICS FOR NURSES** (*Hardy*)

Essentials for **HEALTH PROMOTION IN NURSING**: Promoting Wellness (*Miller*)

Essentials for Nurses About **HOME IN FUSION THERAPY**: The Expert's Best Practice Guide (*Gorski*)

Essentials for the **HOSPICE NURSE**: A Concise Guide to End-of-Life Care, Second Edition (*Wright*)

Essentials about **LGBTQ+ CARE FOR NURSES** (*Traister*)

Essentials for the **LONG-TERM CARE NURSE**: What Nursing Home and Assisted Living Nurses Need to Know (*Eliopoulos*)

Essentials to **LOVING YOUR RESEARCH PROJECT**: A Stress-Free Guide for Novice Researchers in Nursing and Healthcare (*Marshall*)

Essentials for **MAKING THE MOST OF YOUR CAREER IN NURSING** (*Redulla*)

Essentials for **MANAGING PATIENTS WITH APSYCHIATRIC DISORDER**: What RNs, NPs, and New Psych Nurses Need to Know (*Marshall*)

Essentials About **MEDICAL CANNABIS AND OPIOIDS**: Minimizing Opioid Use Through Cannabis (*Smith, Smith*)

Essentials for the **MEDICAL OFFICE NURSE**: What You Really Need to Know (*Richmeier*)

Essentials for the **MEDICAL–SURGICAL NURSE**: Clinical Orientation (*Ciocco*)

Essentials for the **MIDWIVES**: Labor & Delivery Orientation, Third Edition (*Groll*)

Essentials for the **OPERATING ROOM NURSE**, Third Edition (*Criscitelli*)

Essentials for **PATIENT SAFETY IN NURSING**: How to Decrease Medical Errors and Improve Patient Outcomes (*Hunt*)

Essentials for **PSYCHOPHARMACOLOGY FOR NURSE PRACTITIONERS** (*Goldin*)

# *ESSENTIALS* on GENETICS AND GENOMICS FOR NURSES

## Practical Applications

Kimberly A. Subasic, PhD, MS, BSN, CNE

SPRINGER PUBLISHING

Springer Publishing Company, LLC
11 West 42nd Street, New York, NY 10036
www.springerpub.com
connect.springerpub.com/

*Acquisitions Editor: Joseph Morita*
*Compositor*: Transforma

*ISBN*: 978-0-8261-8457-3

Printed by LSI



The *Essentials* series was published in the United States of America as the *Fast Facts* series.

*This book is dedicated to nurses who seek to correlate the future of healthcare and the application of genomics. Proceeds from this book will be given to the International Society of Nurses in Genetics (ISONG). This professional organization comprises nurse researchers, nurse practitioners, and nurse educators who seek to improve healthcare with the utilization of genomic knowledge. The collaborative efforts of nurses in ISONG have led to advances in genomics research, changes to clinical practice, multiple publications and presentations, and the addition of genomics in all levels of nursing education.*

# Contents

# Contributors

**Dhaneesha Bahadur, MSN, RN, LNCC,** Legal Nurse Consultant, Private Practice, New York, New York

**Eric Barbato, PhD, RN,** Assistant Professor, Frances Payne Bolton School of Nursing, Case Western Reserve University, Cleveland, Ohio

**Kathleen A. Calzone, PhD, RN, AGN-BC, FAAN,** Research Geneticist, Genetics Branch, Center for Cancer Research, National Cancer Institute, Bethesda, Maryland

**Dennis J. Cheek, PhD, MSN,** Abell-Hanger Professor of Gerontological Nursing, Harris College of Nursing & Health Sciences, Texas Christian University, Fort Worth, Texas

**Sandra Daack-Hirsch, PhD, RN, FAAN (she, her, hers),** Professor and Executive Associate Dean, College of Nursing, University of Iowa, Iowa City, Iowa

**Caitlin Dreisbach, PhD, RN,** Postdoctoral Research Scientist, Data Science Institute, Columbia University, New York, New York

**Susan C. Grayson, BSN, RN,** Doctoral Student, University of Pittsburgh School of Nursing, Pittsburgh, Pennsylvania

**Michael J. Groves, PhD, RN,** Associate Professor Emeritus, Shepherd University School of Nursing, Shepherdstown, West Virginia

**José de Jesús López Jiménez,** Profesor de Asignatura B, Centro Universitario de Ciencias de la Salud. Departamento de Morfología y Departamento de Disciplinas Filosóficas Metodológicas e

Instrumentales, Universidad de Guadalajara, Guadalajara, México and Centro de Investigación Biomédica de Occidente, Instituto Mexicano del Seguro Social, Guadalajara, Jalisco, México

**Christine (Tina) Mladenka, DNP, APRN, CNP, WHNP-BC,** Nurse Practitioner, Southeastern Idaho Public Health and Adjunct Faculty, Idaho State University, Pocatello, Idaho

**Alexandra Noel Grace,** Instructor and Nurse Practitioner, The Children's Hospital of San Antonio Pediatric Genetics, Baylor College of Medicine, Houston, Texas

**Nico Osier, PhD, RN,** Assistant Professor, University of Texas at Austin School of Nursing and Dell Medical School, Austin, Texas

**Ana Lilia Fletes Rayas,** Profesor Investigador Asociado, Centro Universitario de Ciencias de la Salud, Departamento de Enfermería Clínica Aplicada, Universidad de Guadalajara, Guadalajara, Mexico

**Kathryn Robinson, PhD, MHA/Ed., RN,** Associate Director, Assistant Professor, Jonas Nurse Leader PhD Scholar, School of Nursing, University of Maine, Orono, Maine

**Kim Subasic, PhD, MS, BSN, CNE,** Assistant Professor and Department Head, Swain Department of Nursing, The Citadel, Charleston, South Carolina

**Deborah Tamura,** Research Nurse, Laboratory of Cancer Biology and Genetics, Center for Cancer Research, National Cancer Institute, National Institutes of Health, Bethesda, Maryland

**McKenzie K. Wallace, PhD, RN,** Assistant Professor, The Ohio State University, College of Nursing, Columbus, Ohio

**Susan W. Wesmiller, PhD, RN, FAAN,** Associate Professor, Genomics Hub, Health, Promotion and Development, School of Nursing, University of Pittsburgh, Pittsburgh, Pennsylvania

# Preface

The purpose of this book is to provide readers with an introduction to genetics and genomics, and how this knowledge is applied in the clinical setting. Each chapter addresses how healthcare has been impacted by genomics and its implications in practice. Rapid advances in genomics have changed clinical expectations and the utilization of genomics in the care of the patient and the family. It is imperative that nurses have genomic knowledge that can be implemented into clinical practice. Nurse educators must be adept at teaching genomic content throughout a nursing curriculum, and at every degree level. Nurses will be held accountable for the application of genomics in the assessment and treatment of the patient. Considerations of how genetics impacts the family and subsequent care will be an added expectation. Nurses must have genomic knowledge so they can advocate for patient and family care as part of the delivery of personalized healthcare, and in the utilization of genomic advances to improve patient outcomes. The broad range of genetic concepts provided in this book offers foundational knowledge of genetics and genomics that can be immediately applied in a teaching or clinical setting.

# 1

# Introduction to Genetics and Genomics

Caitlin Dreisbach

*As nurses, we all learned in our required coursework about deoxyribonucleic acid, or DNA, as our primary heredity material. Genetics, or the study of our hereditary material, is not a new concept to us. Still, how we are using our knowledge of DNA in healthcare has changed dramatically over the last several decades. This chapter provides a history of the exploration of our genetic code, key definitions, and an introduction to the basic units of DNA. Subsequent chapters in this book will build from the knowledge learned here and walk you through a comprehensive understanding of how we can use genetics to better inform the care of our patients.*

**In this chapter, you will learn:**

1. A brief history of how we have come to understand our genetic code
2. The introductory definitions for genetics and genomic concepts
3. The fundamentals of DNA structure and function

## A HISTORY OF OUR DNA

Genetics, or the study of our heredity material, has been observed for thousands of years, but it first emerged with rigorous and scientific investigation through the work of Gregor Mendel. Mendel was a 19th-century monk examining the patterns of inheritance of specific traits in pea plants (Miko, 2008). By observing, recording, and testing how specific patterns are passed along the generations of the peas, Mendel identified the unit of inheritance that we now know as a gene. Genes are the basic units of heredity and are composed of smaller chemical bases in deoxyribonucleic acid, or DNA. Genes give instructions to make molecules, called proteins, which are essential for the body to perform crucial functions in relation to our health and well-being.

The modern study of genetics has moved beyond recording inheritance patterns to diving deeper into the molecular structure of genes, including how they function in expected and pathological health states. The advancement of genetics occurred when Rosalind Franklin, a British chemist, was the first to visualize the structure of the DNA molecule using x-ray crystallography (Klug, 1968). Her chemical understanding of DNA, and subsequent picture evidence of the molecule, was shared with Francis Crick and James Watson, two scientists at Cambridge University. Watson and Crick then widely disseminated that DNA was made up of two chains of nucleotide pairs, with a sugar and phosphate backbone, that account for the genetic material of all living beings. Some accounts claim that Watson and Crick gained their popularity and status by using the work of Rosalind Franklin without giving her appropriate credit.

In 2003, the completion of the Human Genome Project (HGP) exploded a new age of genetic inquiry. The HGP was an international collaboration seeking to understand all of the genes in humans, also known as our **genome** (National Human Genome Research Institute, 2018). The results of the research found that there are approximately 20,500 genes in the human body. By identifying and understanding the structure of each of these genes, more recent work on personalized health and genomic-informed care has grown. Concurrent discussions about the ethical and social implications of the HGP are still being documented. Because of the significant advancements in technology and in our understanding of how genes work in health and disease, new information about our genetics continues to appear in clinical practice settings.

**Essential Facts**

The Human Genome Project advanced the study of genetics by mapping all the genes in the human body.

## KEY DEFINITIONS

Definitions for key terms that lay the foundation of genetics and genomics in this book are presented in Table 1.1. More terms will be provided throughout subsequent chapters to supplement this list.

Table 1.1

**Vocabulary**

| Term | Definition |
|---|---|
| Gene | Basic unit of heredity, composed of DNA |
| Genotype | Set of alleles at a particular gene location |
| Genetics | The study of individual genes and their impact on health and well-being |
| Genomics | The study of all the genes in the human body, including gene interactions with the environment, and psychosocial and cultural factors |
| DNA | Deoxyribonucleic acid; molecule arranged in a double-helix structure that is responsible for the instructions for cell development, growth, and reproduction |
| RNA | Ribonucleic acid; a single-stranded molecule responsible for gene expression |
| Protein | A molecule made up of amino acids for a particular function in the human body |
| Alleles | Different versions of a gene, typically there are two or more |
| Nitrogenous base | In DNA, the four bases are adenine (A), thymine (T), cytosine (C), and guanine (G). In RNA, uracil (U) replaces thymine |
| Codon | A set of three consecutive nitrogenous bases |
| Amino acids | Building blocks of a protein |
| Chromosomes | Molecular structures within the nucleus that carry DNA |
| Transcription | The process of creating RNA to direct protein synthesis |
| Translation | The process of creating proteins that occur after transcription |
| Mutation | A change in one or more genes |
| Phenotype | Observable characteristic |

## DNA STRUCTURE

DNA is arranged in a helical structure with two backbone strands winding around each other. Similar to a spiral staircase, the strands wrap around each other in a design called a double helix. The strands are linked together by nitrogenous bases, or the basic chemical building blocks of DNA. The nitrogenous bases are chemically bonded together and have a specific pattern of linkage. The four types of bases in DNA are adenine (A), thymine (T), cytosine (C), and guanine (G). The bases have specific pairs that attract each other in a pattern of adenine and thymine (A and T) and cytosine and guanine (C and G). Figure 1.1 shows a simplified version of DNA. The backbone of the DNA helix is composed of sugar and phosphate chemical groups. These sugar and phosphate groups support the nitrogenous bases as they link the strands. The backbone is oriented from 5' to 3', a notation for the direction and orientation of the DNA strand. The opposite orientation of the strands is called antiparallelism.

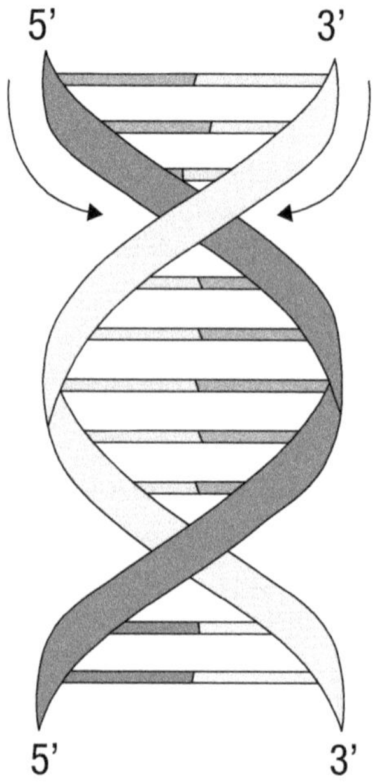


**Figure 1.1** The structure of DNA in a double helix. The figure illustrates the double-stranded helix structure oriented from the 5′ to 3′ end. The multicolored linkages between the strands represent the nitrogenous bases.

**Essential Facts**

The DNA molecule is shaped in a double helix with a backbone of sugar and phosphate groups that are linked together by nitrogenous bases.

## THE CENTRAL DOGMA AND THE FUNCTION OF DNA

The underlying theory of genetic information transfer is called the Central Dogma. The Central Dogma states that genetic information flows from DNA to RNA and then to a protein. **RNA**, or ribonucleic acid, is a molecule similar to DNA. It has a similar phosphate and sugar backbone (DNA has deoxyribose, and RNA has ribose as the sugar), but it is only single stranded. RNA does not have thymine as a nitrogenous base. Instead, thymine is replaced by uracil. Uracil is then paired with adenine, just as the thymine is in DNA. First shared by Francis Crick, the Central Dogma provided a groundwork for thinking about genes expressing information from DNA through transcription and translation. We will review a simplified version of these foundational processes in this section.

As you recall from the previous section, the DNA molecule is made up of nitrogenous bases that pair and link the backbone strands. Each set of three consecutive nitrogenous bases is called a **codon**. A codon gives instructions for the creation of an **amino acid**, the building blocks of proteins. Genes comprise a specific number of codons that, in combination, provide comprehensive instructions for protein manufacturing.

To get all the information from within the cell's nucleus, the DNA must first be replicated. In DNA replication, the backbone strands of the DNA unwind and separate from each other, leaving single strands available for transcription. The process of transcription copies the base sequence of the separated single DNA strand and makes a new molecule called messenger RNA (mRNA). The new mRNA molecule then undergoes translation, the process by which proteins are synthesized from the particular amino acid sequence. The result of completing both transcription and translation is the creation of a protein.

## GENETICS, THE HUMAN BODY, AND DISEASE

Each gene has one or more alternative forms, called **alleles**, found at the exact location on a chromosome. A child receives a maternal and a paternal allele on 23 chromosomes during reproduction. A **chromosome** is a structure within the nucleus of a cell that carries DNA. In total, humans typically have 46 chromosomes (23 from each parent). The chromosomes in the twenty-third pair are called the sex chromosomes and are primarily responsible for human sex. Females have two copies of an X chromosome (one from the mother and one from the father), and males have an X and a Y (the X from the mother and the Y from the father). There are chromosomal disorders in which an individual has a different number of total chromosomes than 46, such as Turner syndrome, where a female is partially or entirely missing an X chromosome (45 chromosomes total), or Down syndrome, where a child gets an extra twenty-first chromosome (47 chromosomes total).

A variation that arises from a **mutation** in the genetic sequence for each allele means that the gene still codes for the same trait, but it is expressed differently. Mutations are changes in the genetic code. Mutations can be harmful or might represent the variation across humans. An example of allelic variation that is not harmful is blood type. The classification of blood type is based on the alleles given from each parent during reproduction. There are three possible alleles for the gene that expresses blood type: A, B, and O. The **genotype**, or set of alleles at a particular gene location, dictates which blood type is expressed. The final expressed blood type is called the **phenotype**, or the observable characteristic of the genotype. An individual with A blood type has a genotype of AA or AO compared to someone with B blood type with a genotype of BB or BO.

Unexpected changes can happen anywhere in the production of a protein. A change in the gene can alter which type of protein is created or if there is even a protein synthesized at all. An example of a mutation that alters the production of a protein occurs in Duchenne Muscular Dystrophy (DMD). In patients with DMD, a gene mutation results in a decreased amount of the protein dystrophin being synthesized in the body. Dystrophin is responsible for supporting muscle contraction. Without it, muscles cannot efficiently contract and support the movement, because fibrous tissue replaces healthy muscle. Patients with DMD have progressive muscle damage and weakness, often beginning in early childhood. There is variation in the mutation at the *DMD* gene in which some patients produce virtually zero dystrophin protein and others make enough to be functional. The amount of protein that is produced commands the severity of the disease. Not all gene mutations cause a functional change in the protein, so linking diseases to single mutations can be challenging. In most cases, diseases are a combination of genetic modification, the environment, and other factors happening in the body. The variety of factors that cause symptoms or disease are called multifactorial conditions compared to a condition caused by a single gene mutation, a Mendelian condition.

**Essential Facts**

Diseases that are caused by a combination of genetics and the environment are called multifactorial conditions.

## RELEVANCE TO NURSING

Nurses have a direct role in the communication of genetic and genomic information. Whether caring for a patient with a known genetic disorder or assisting a family with getting access to genetic testing, nurses are critical liaisons between advancing technology, genetic knowledge, and the care of patients. In 2008, a consensus panel convened to determine the minimum competencies needed to prepare the nursing workforce to deliver genomic-informed care (Consensus Panel, 2008). The resulting document, titled "Essentials of Genetic and Genomic Nursing: Competencies, Curricula Guidelines, and Outcome Indicators," outlined the professional responsibilities of nurses in the domain of genetics and genomics. According to the "Essentials" documentation, nurses should be able to apply and integrate genetic information through their knowledge base, patient assessment, provision of education, and plan of care development. As nurses, it is within our scope of practice to facilitate referrals to other specialized genetic and genomic services, including counseling and genetic testing. Finally, nurses should be capable of assessing the impact and effectiveness of genetic and genomic interventions and treatments on the health outcomes of our patients.

As technology advances, allowing us to better understand the human genome, our knowledge of the application of genetics and genomics to patient care is changing. Personalized health, or the use of a patient's genomic information to make more accurate and individualized decisions, is unfolding rapidly. Technology, such as CRISPR, which is used to edit specific genes, has the great potential of drastically changing the way modern medicine approaches patients with a genetic disorder. More discussion about the ethical and social implications of gene-editing technology will be discussed in later chapters of this book.

**Essential Facts**

Genetic and genomic technology is rapidly advancing and has the potential to change patient health outcomes substantially.

## END-OF-CHAPTER QUESTIONS

1. Name three ways that the Human Genome Project advanced healthcare.
2. Give an example of a Mendelian condition and of a multifactorial condition. Explain the genetic contribution to each condition.
3. Order the following terms that you learned in this section from the smallest to the largest: genome, nucleotide base pairs, chromosome, gene, and DNA.
4. What is included in the role of the nurses when it comes to taking care of patients with a genetic disorder?
   A. Referring patients and their families to genetic counseling services.
   B. Reviewing their medications for potential genetic interactions.
   C. Supporting patients during prenatal genetic testing.
   D. Offering educational materials on a genetic condition.
   E. All of the above

## VIGNETTE

A nurse admits an 8-year-old patient to the pediatric unit for worsening lung function who is diagnosed with cystic fibrosis (CF). The nurse remembers that CF is a genetic condition but wants to learn more to best care for the patient. After he completes the patient's physical assessment and provides the necessary care, the nurse uses MedlinePlus to get more information about the disease. He finds out that there is a wide variation in symptom severity and disease progression for CF. He reviews his patient's medical record and finds out that the patient previously received genetic testing. The nurse sees that the patient's testing reveals that his alleles for the cystic fibrosis transmembrane conductance regulator (CFTR) gene are some of the most severe. The nurse recalls from his coursework that the specific genotype dictates the extent of expressed phenotype. Knowing this information, the nurse can anticipate the potential for needing more advanced care for this patient and communicates that to his charge nurse.

## REFERENCES

Consensus Panel. (2008). *Essentials of genetic and genomic nursing: Competencies, curricula guidelines, and outcome indicators* (2nd ed., pp. 1–80). American Nurses Association.

Klug, A. (1968). Rosalind Franklin and the discovery of the structure of DNA. *Nature, 219*(5156), 808–810. https://doi.org/10.1038/219808a0

Miko, I. (2008). Gregor Mendel and the principles of inheritance. *Nature Education, 1*(1), 134.

National Human Genome Research Institute. (2018). *What is the Human Genome Project?* Genome.gov. https://www.genome.gov/human-genome-project/What

# 2

# Gene Expression

McKenzie K. Wallace and Eric Barbato

*In Chapter 1, we learned the basics of what a gene is—a hereditary unit of DNA that encodes a functional product, most often a protein. But what about the steps in between DNA and its protein? What becomes of a protein after it has been made? What controls when a protein is made? The answers to these questions make up the topic of this chapter: gene expression.*

**In this chapter, you will learn:**

1. The relationship between genotype and phenotype
2. Mechanisms that control gene expression
3. The relationship between inherited alleles and gene expression

## BASICS OF GENE EXPRESSION

Gene expression is the method by which a gene is used to make its product, which then makes an observable effect in a lifeform. As we learned in Chapter 1, this process is known today as the central dogma of genetics: DNA makes RNA makes protein. The aforementioned observable effect exerted by a gene is known as a phenotype. Gene products such as proteins can affect phenotype in many ways, some more apparent than others. It is important to note that while humans all share the same chromosomes and the same genes, the sequence of those genes varies greatly between people of different sexes and ethnicities. This variation in our DNA is what makes us so diverse in phenotype.

The different forms of a gene possessed by different people (due to variation in their DNA) are called **alleles**. As you may remember from previous chapters, under normal circumstances, we each inherit two copies of every gene, that is to say, two alleles: one from our biological mother and one from our biological father. The combination of these two alleles for all the genetic material in our bodies defines our genotype. It should be noted, however, that when people say "genotype" they are most often referring to a single locus or set of loci in the genome. For example, an individual with cystic fibrosis possesses two copies of the CFTR gene, both of which feature a disease-causing mutation. A clinician might refer to those mutations as that individual's "CFTR genotype" or "genotype for CFTR."

**Essential Facts**

- An allele is a version of a gene; every person has two copies of every gene, but the alleles of that gene they have may be different.
- The pair of alleles someone has is called their genotype.

## FROM DNA TO PROTEIN

We've covered the basic concept of gene expression and how it ultimately affects phenotype, but what are the steps a gene takes to eventually become a protein? The answer was first described by Francis Crick in his 1957 manuscript, *On protein synthesis*. In that work, Dr. Crick laid out the central dogma of genetics: DNA makes RNA makes protein. We now know that some genes have products other than proteins, but most genes in our DNA conform to this standard.

To begin its journey to become a protein, DNA must first make RNA, a process known as transcription. Transcription is facilitated in the nucleus of our cells by an enzyme called polymerase that binds to DNA, moving along the length of the DNA strand and synthesizing a new strand of complementary RNA. There are many types of RNA, but the type that is the product of transcription is called messenger RNA or mRNA. After mRNA is formed, it carries its message outside of the nucleus to an organelle called the ribosome, where protein is made.

Once the mRNA is bound, the ribosome then binds another type of RNA called transfer RNA or tRNA. tRNA is a specialized molecule that serves to read the message carried by mRNA in groups of three nucleotide bases at a time—these tri-nucleotide groups are called **codons** (Sharp et al., 1985). As it reads the message, tRNA begins stringing together a chain of protein building blocks called **amino acids** (Crick et al., 1961). This process of creating a chain of amino acids from mRNA is called **translation**. Once the entire message has been read and the corresponding amino acids have been chained together, the result is a complete protein. It should be noted that many proteins undergo certain changes after they have been synthesized at the ribosome. This process, known as post-translational modification, is one of the many tools our bodies use to produce diverse proteins from relatively few different amino acids.

## THE GENETIC CODE

Now that we have reviewed the process by which DNA produces a protein, let's explore a few of the important differences between DNA, RNA, and protein. As we covered in Chapter 1, DNA is made up of four nucleotide bases: A (adenine), C (cytosine), T (thymine), and G (guanine). DNA forms its signature double-helix structure by following a simple pairing rule: A pairs with T, and C pairs with G. Herein lie the two most important differences between DNA and RNA. RNA also features four nucleotide bases, but replaces thymine with **U (uracil)**, making its four bases A, C, U, and G. Additionally, RNA only occurs naturally in single-stranded form, meaning that its bases are not paired as in DNA. This quality makes RNA a comparatively unstable molecule.

As mentioned earlier in this chapter, each tri-nucleotide codon encodes one of 20 different amino acids. Some codons even encode the same amino acid. For example, the codon AGC encodes the amino acid serine, and GGG encodes glycine, though TCA also encodes serine. There are, however, two important exceptions to this rule.

A gene must have a way to tell the molecular machinery responsible for transcription and translation where the gene starts and stops. There are a few special codons that encode the genetic instructions for START and STOP. The codon ATG (or AUG in mRNA), for example, encodes the amino acid methionine, which instructs the ribosome to start translating everything that comes after it. Once the ribosome has translated all of the subsequent message, the codons TAA, TAG, and TGA encode the instructions for the ribosome to stop translation. With these exceptions, all other tri-nucleotide combinations encode an amino acid.

**Essential Facts**

- A codon is a functional group of three nucleotides that encodes an amino acid.
- The human genome encodes 20 amino acids, which are the building blocks of the proteins in our bodies.

## GENOMIC REGULATION OF GENE EXPRESSION

The genome contained within our cells' nuclei is made up of 3.2 billion base pairs that encode about 20,000 discrete genes. The proteins that make up the diverse tissues in our bodies, however, are far more numerous. So, how is it possible that a library of only 20,000 genes can produce well over a million different proteins? Our bodies have a few ways to get around this problem; one of the most important to this chapter is called splicing.

You may remember from Chapter 1 that a gene is functionally divided into many parts, two of which are exons, which encode protein, and **introns**, which contain instructions for where, when, and in what amount a protein should be expressed (Gilbert, 1978). When a gene is transcribed into mRNA, it undergoes a process called splicing in which the introns are removed, leaving only the exons packed next to one another. For example, a gene containing four exons may be spliced in such a way that all four exons are present in the following order: 1 – 2 – 3 – 4. Genes vary greatly in length—some have only a few exons, and some have dozens. However, when a gene is spliced, not all of the exons may be present in the mRNA product. The same four-exon gene may be spliced in such a way that the resulting mRNA contains only three exons in the following orders: 1 – 3 – 4 or 1 – 2 – 4. Since proteins are made up of amino acids in a specific order, the mRNA that only contains exons 1, 2, and 4 will produce a different protein than the mRNA that contains exons 1, 3, and 4. Meanwhile, both of those proteins will be different than the one produced by the mRNA that contains all four exons. This process is called **alternative splicing** and is one of the main ways our bodies are able to synthesize so many proteins from so few genes.

**Essential Facts**

- The human genome encodes about 20,000 discrete genes, yet produces hundreds of thousands of different proteins.
- Alternative splicing is a method by which one gene can encode many proteins.

## EPIGENOMIC REGULATION OF GENE EXPRESSION

Simply stated, the **epigenome** is a set of modifications to DNA that play a critical role in regulating gene expression. Our bodies are made up of many different cell types, such as skin cells and muscle cells. Though cells differ in form and function, each cell in our bodies has the same genome in its nucleus. Epigenetic modification of that genome is what directs cell differentiation in the embryo, instructing your cells to become smooth muscle cells in your intestines or epithelial cells in your skin (Handy et al., 2011). Numerous mechanisms exist that regulate and change the epigenome, and thus control gene expression. Two of the most important mechanisms of epigenetic regulation that have an effect on gene expression are DNA methylation and histone modification (Moore et al., 2013; Stillman, 2018).

As you'll recall from Chapter 1, our genomes are incredibly large—about 3.2 billion base pairs long. To accommodate the enormous size of our genome, our DNA is organized into packages called **nucleosomes**. Nucleosomes are units of DNA that are wrapped around organizing proteins called **histones** (Handy et al., 2011). This collection of nucleosomes makes up a substance called **chromatin**, which then organizes into 23 chromosome pairs. Histones can be modified to facilitate the expression (or "turning on") of our genes. When it is time for a cell to make a specific protein, the DNA encoding only that protein can be unraveled, transcribed, and translated, rather than unwinding the entire genetic code.

Histones can be modified, resulting in DNA's being more tightly wound (condensed chromatin structure) or more loosely wound (loose or active chromatin structure). When DNA is tightly wound it cannot be easily read by transcription enzymes, thus the gene will not be expressed. Each histone has a tail region that can be modified. Modification of this tail can cause the entire chromatin structure to be more tightly or loosely wound, affecting the expression of the associated genes (Stillman, 2018). Histone modification plays an important role in cancer development. Histone modification can lead to overexpression of oncogenes—cancer-causing genes—or suppress the expression of tumor-suppressor genes (Stillman, 2018), both of which are processes commonly found in cancer development (Audia and Campbell, 2016).

Another important mechanism of epigenetic modification involves "turning off" certain genes. This process, called **DNA methylation**, is the addition of a methyl group to a specific site in our DNA, which renders the associated DNA unreadable by transcription enzymes, thereby preventing gene expression. Methylation only happens at certain loci in the genome called CpG **sites**, so named for the two nucleotides involved: cytosine (C) and guanine (G), between which lies the backbone of DNA structure—phosphate (p) (Handy et al., 2011). During embryo development, most CpG sites are methylated as part of stem cell differentiation and other developmental processes (Handy et al., 2011). This type of methylation is critical for normal development and function in humans. This methylation is considered stable and inherited, meaning it will stay the same throughout an individual's life (Handy et al., 2011).

A small number of CpG sites exist in the DNA that are typically unmethylated—these are referred to as CpG islands (Moore et al., 2013). Many of these CpG islands are located in the promoter region of genes, and thus can exert an effect on DNA transcription and gene expression (Handy et al., 2011). The majority of research on DNA methylation in the context of human disease is focused on these CpG islands, since the default is for these regions to be unmethylated (Moore et al., 2013). We often refer to methylation in terms of "hypermethylation," meaning many methyl groups are present, and "hypomethylation," meaning few methyl groups are present. The physiologic outcome of methylation depends on the function of the gene. For example, if a proto-oncogene is hypomethylated, meaning the gene is more likely to be expressed (or "turned on"), a tumor can grow, leading to cancer. Similarly, if a tumor-suppressor gene is hypermethylated, meaning the gene is less likely to be expressed, a cancer-causing growth can also develop (Lim & Maher, 2010).

CpGs can become hypermethylated or hypomethylated due to environmental exposures like air pollution, smoking, metabolic dysfunction (obesity), diet, stress, physical activity, and so forth (Martin & Fry, 2018). This methylation is dynamic and can change throughout a person's life, leading to differences in gene expression across the lifespan and ultimately contributing to disease (Martin & Fry, 2018). Understanding and quantifying the impact of environmental factors and social and behavioral determinants of health on methylation is a high priority of nursing research.

## Essential Facts

- Methylation influences the readability of DNA by adding methyl groups to cytosine nucleotides, making it difficult for transcription enzymes to reach the DNA.
- Histone modification changes how tightly wound the DNA is, with tightly wound DNA being inaccessible to be read and loosely wound DNA being ready for transcription.

## ALLELIC IMBALANCES

Differences in gene expression can also result from allelic imbalances. Every individual inherits two copies of every allele, a paternal copy and a maternal copy. Normally, each allele is expressed, and the phenotype depends on the inheritance pattern for that gene. However, in some instances, only one allele is expressed. This is called monoallelic expression (Singer-Sam, 2010). In cases of monoallelic expression, only one allele is expressed, either the maternal or the paternal allele, and the other allele is hypermethylated, making the DNA from one allele inaccessible and thus not transcribed (Eckersley-Maslin & Spector, 2014; Singer-Sam, 2010).

Imprinting is one type of monoallelic expression. Across the genome, there are a handful of genes that are expressed either from the paternal line or from the maternal line (Lobo, 2008). One example is insulinlike growth factor 2 *(IGF2)*. *IGF2* is always expressed from the paternal line, while the maternal copy is hypermethylated, preventing expression (Bergman et al., 2013).

In most cases, imprinting is a normal process that does not result in adverse phenotypes. However, if there is a mutation in the only active allele, an abnormal phenotype can be the result. The most common genetic disorders associated with imprinting are Prader–Willi Syndrome and Angelman Syndrome. In both syndromes, the same portion of chromosome 15 is missing, but the phenotype depends on the parental origin of chromosome deletion (Butler et al., 2019; Margolis et al., 2015). In Prader–Willi Syndrome, the deletion is inherited from the father, resulting in a lack of expression of the *SNRPN* and *NDN* genes (Butler et al., 2019). Prader–Willi Syndrome is characterized by poor muscle tone and increased appetite in childhood that often leads to extreme obesity. Individuals with Prader–Willi Syndrome often also exhibit intellectual disability and behavioral changes. As with most genetic syndromes, certain characteristic physical changes are associated with Prader–Willi Syndrome, including a narrow forehead, almond shaped eyes, triangular mouth, small hands and feet, and underdeveloped genitalia (Butler et al., 2019). Conversely, Angelman Syndrome results when the missing portion of chromosome 15 is inherited from the mother, resulting in a lack of expression of the *UBE3A* gene. Angelman Syndrome is associated with a different phenotype, defined by several development delays and intellectual disabilities, as well as hyperactivity and a reduced need for sleep (Margolis et al., 2015).

**X inactivation** is another, necessary, type of monoallelic expression. Typically, females inherit two X chromosomes while males inherit one X chromosome and one Y chromosome. Females do not need all of the information from both X chromosomes; indeed, expression of the entirety of both X chromosomes would lead to deleterious effects. Therefore, early in embryonic development, in each individual cell, one of the X chromosomes is inactivated, permanently preventing expression of nearly every locus on that chromosome (Disteche & Berletch, 2015). This process occurs in early development and is entirely random. Some cells may silence the paternal X chromosome while others silence the maternal X chromosome. Since the inactivation process is entirely random, in general, about 50% of a female's cells will have the paternal X chromosome active and about 50% will have the maternal X chromosome active (Disteche & Berletch, 2015). However, skewed X chromosome inactivation can occur, in which case 70% or more of an individual's expressed X-chromosome may come from one parent (Shvetsova et al., 2019). If no mutations are present, no issues will occur. But if the skewed inactivation results in more of the X chromosome coming from a parent with an X-linked recessive trait, like hemophilia, then the greater expression of the mutated gene from the X chromosome may result in the individual's having some clinical symptoms of the condition, but this is incredibly rare (Shoukat et al., 2020). Skewed X inactivation may lead to delays in diagnosis of X-linked conditions given the rarity of such outcomes and due to the presence of some normally functioning genes, leading to less severe clinical presentations (Shoukat et al., 2020; Shvetsova et al., 2019).

**Essential Facts**

- Imprinting refers to inactivation of the allele from one parent so that only one parental allele is expressed at specific gene loci based on predetermined inheritance patterns.
- X inactivation is a process that takes place in females to "silence" portions of the X chromosome inherited from each parent so females only express one X chromosome, with approximately half from the father and half from the mother.

## CONCLUSION

The complex interaction between epigenetics and genetics is highly relevant to nursing care. Epigenomic dysregulation is strongly implicated in the development of numerous cancers, and is a cause of the heterogeneity observed within cancer phenotypes. Genetic testing of tumors is quickly becoming standard to identify the best course of treatment from the outset. Epigenetic changes also have implications for almost every human disease given that environmental, social, and behavioral factors can also lead to changes in methylation, which can lead to disease. Understanding the epigenetic contributions to disease is important for providing patients with information to make decisions about how they will approach their health.

## END-OF-CHAPTER QUESTIONS

1. What is the difference between genotype and phenotype?
2. What are two major differences between RNA and DNA?
3. What is the difference between transcription and translation?
4. What is the difference between an exon and an intron?
5. How is it that our bodies can produce multiple proteins from the same gene?
6. How can lifestyle behaviors or environmental exposures contribute to gene expression?
7. What are two major epigenetic methods of gene expression regulation?

## REFERENCES

Audia, J. E., & Campbell, R. M. (2016). Histone modifications and cancer. *Cold Spring Harbor Perspectives in Biology, 8*(4), a019521. https://doi.org/10.1101/cshperspect.a019521

Bergman, D., Halje, M., Nordin, M., & Engström, W. (2013). Insulin-like growth factor 2 in development and disease: A mini-review. *Gerontology, 59*(3), 240–249. https://doi.org/10.1159/000343995

Butler, M. G., Miller, J. L., & Forster, J. L. (2019). Prader–Willi syndrome – Clinical genetics, diagnosis and treatment approaches: An update. *Current Pediatric Reviews, 15*(4), 207–244. https://doi.org/10.2174/1573396315666190716120925

Crick, F., Barnett, L., Brenner, S., & Watts-Tobin, R. J. (1961). General nature of the genetic code for proteins. *Nature, 92*, 1227–1232.

Disteche, C. M., & Berletch, J. B. (2015). X-chromosome inactivation and escape. *Journal of Genetics, 94*(4), 591–599. https://doi.org/10.1007/s12041-015-0574-1

Eckersley-Maslin, M. A., & Spector, D. L. (2014). Random monoallelic expression: Regulating gene expression one allele at a time. *Trends in Genetics, 30*(6), 237–244. https://doi.org/10.1016/j.tig.2014.03.003

Gilbert, W. (1978). Why genes in pieces? *Nature, 271*(5645), 501–501.

Handy, D. E., Castro, R., & Loscalzo, J. (2011). Epigenetic modifications: Basic mechanisms and role in cardiovascular disease. *Circulation, 123*(19), 2145–2156. https://doi.org/10.1161/circulationaha.110.956839

Lim, D. H., & Maher, E. R. (2010). DNA methylation: A form of epigenetic control of gene expression. *Obstetrician & Gynaecologist, 12*(1), 37–42.

Lobo, I. (2008). Genomic imprinting and patterns of disease inheritance. *Nature Education, 1*(1), 66. https://www.nature.com/scitable/topicpage/genomic-imprinting-and-patterns-of-disease-inheritance-899/

Margolis, S. S., Sell, G. L., Zbinden, M. A., & Bird, L. M. (2015). Angelman syndrome. *Neurotherapeutics, 12*(3), 641–650. https://doi.org/10.1007/s13311-015-0361-y

Martin, E. M., & Fry, R. C. (2018). Environmental influences on the epigenome: Exposure-associated DNA methylation in human populations. *Annual Review of Public Health, 39*, 309–333. https://doi.org/10.1146/annurev-publhealth-040617-014629

Moore, L. D., Le, T., & Fan, G. (2013). DNA methylation and its basic function. *Neuropsychopharmacology, 38*(1), 23–38. https://doi.org/10.1038/npp.2012.112

Sharp, S. J., Schaack, J., Cooley, L., Burke, D. J., & Soil, D. (1985). Structure and transcription of eukaryotic tRNA gene. *Critical Reviews in Biochemistry, 19*(2), 107–144.

Shoukat, H. M. H., Ghous, G., Tarar, Z. I., Shoukat, M. M., & Ajmal, N. (2020). Skewed inactivation of X chromosome: A cause of hemophilia manifestation in carrier females. *Cureus, 12*(10).

Shvetsova, E., Sofronova, A., Monajemi, R., Gagalova, K., Draisma, H. H. M., White, S. J., Santen, G. W. E., Chuva de Sousa Lopes, S. M., Heijmans, B. T., van Meurs, J., Jansen, R., Franke, L., Kiełbasa, S. M., den Dunnen, J. T., & 't Hoen, P. A. C. (2019). Skewed X-inactivation is common in the general female population. *European Journal of Human Genetics, 27*(3), 455–465. https://doi.org/10.1038/s41431-018-0291-3

Singer-Sam, J. (2010). Monoallelic expression. *Nature Education, 3*(3), 1. https://www.nature.com/scitable/topicpage/monoallelic-expression-8813275/

Stillman, B. (2018). Histone modifications: Insights into their influence on gene expression. *Cell, 175*(1), 6–9. https://doi.org/10.1016/j.cell.2018.08.032cancer phenotypes

# 3

# Medical Family History

Sandra Daack-Hirsch

*A positive family history of complex diseases such as cancer and type 2 diabetes (T2D) reflects inherited genetic susceptibility as well as shared environmental, cultural, and behavioral factors that increase one's risk for developing it. Hence, family history (familial risk) is used to assess genetic/genomic risk for inherited as well as complex diseases. Accurate assessment and effective communication of familial risk enhances risk stratification (Audrain-McGovern et al., 2003; Yoon et al., 2003), allowing nurses to reassure those at background -population risk and to discuss screening and treatment options or behavior changes for those with increased risk. Family history is also routinely used to determine who might benefit from genetic testing and in the interpretation of genetic test results. In the United States, affected individuals are largely responsible for notifying at-risk family members of their disease risk so they can be screened and treated. Further, one of the primary reasons for genetic and clinical testing of at-risk relatives is to provide better surveillance of asymptomatic family members across the life span.*

**In this chapter, you will learn:**

1. Benefits of taking a family history in healthcare practice
2. How to create a three-generation pedigree using standard symbols
3. How to identify genomic red flags

## FAMILY HEALTH HISTORY

Your knowledge of your patient's family health history can aid in the diagnosis and treatment of rare single-gene disorders such as cystic fibrosis, sickle cell amimia, Huntington's disease, or inherited cancer syndromes. Affected individuals with a known genetic mutation are largely responsible for notifying at-risk family members of their disease risk so they can be screened and treated. Screening of at-risk family members is conducted through cascade screening, a process of sequentially testing at-risk family members through genetic testing and clinical exam. However, identifying at-risk family members is done by collecting a family history. Importantly, family history is a primary risk factor for many chronic diseases, such as type 2 diabeties (T2D), cancer, and heart disease. As such, it is used to promote risk assessment and stratification so that appropriate interventions can occur (Scheuner, 2004). Taking a family history is patient centered and collaborative and can build rapport with patients.

**Essential Facts**

Since 2004, the U.S. Surgeon General has declared Thanksgiving Day as National Family Health History Day. This move was to encourage families to discuss their health histories on a day when everyone catches up.

### Standard Pedigree Symbols

Family health histories are collected and depicted in the form of a pedigree. In short, you solicit family health information and, using a system of standardized symbols and nomenclature (Bennett et al., 2008), create a graphic of families' medical history. Standard pedigree symbols are found in Exhibit 3.1. Symbols for phenotypic gender include a square for males and a circle for females. A diamond is used for persons with gender not specified, a congenital disorder of sex development, with transgendered individuals, or when it is not clinically relevant to assign a gender (Bennett et al., 2008). For transgender and gender-nonconforming people whose gender identity may differ from their phenotypic gender, it could be important to depict their gender identity and denote their biological sex as well (Bennett et al., 2008; Sheehan et al., 2020). For example, when tracking a family history for cancer of reproductive organs, the phenotypic gender is important. Horizontal lines denote mating/partnered relationships, while vertical lines show lines of descent and intergenerational relationships. For more detailed nomenclature see Bennett et al. (2008) and Sheenan et al. (2020) (Exhibit 3.2).

## Exhibit 3.1 Pedigree Symbols

| | Male | Female | Gender not specified | Comments |
|---|---|---|---|---|
| 1. Individual | b. 1925 | 30y | 4 mo | Assign gender by phenotype (see text for disorders of sex development, etc.). Do not write age in symbol. |
| 2. Affected individual | | | | Key/legend used to define shading or other fill (e.g., hatches, dots, etc.). Use only when individual is clinically affected. |
| | | | With ≥2 conditions, the individual's symbol can be partitioned accordingly, each segment shaded with a different fill and defined in legend. | |
| 3. Multiple individuals, number known | 5 | 5 | 5 | Number of siblings written inside symbol. (Affected individuals should not be grouped). |
| 4. Multiple individuals, number unknown or unstated | n | n | n | "n" used in place of "?". |
| 5. Deceased individual | d. 35 | d. 4 mo | d. 60's | Indicate cause of death if known. Do not use a cross (†) to indicates death to avoid confusion with evaluation positive (+). |
| 6. Consultand | | | | Individual(s) seeking genetic counseling/ testing. |
| 7. Proband | P | P | | An affected family member coming to medical attention independent of other family members. |
| 8. Stillbirth (SB) | SB 28 wk | SB 30 wk | SB 34 wk | Include gestational age and karyotype, if known. |
| 9. Pregnancy (P) | P LMP 7/1/2007 47,XY, +21 | P 20 wk 46,XX | P | Gestational age and karyotype below symbol. Light shading can be used for affected; define in key/legend. |

| Pregnancies not carried to term | Affected | Unaffected | |
|---|---|---|---|
| 10. Spontaneous abortion (SAB) | 17 wks female cystic hygroma | < 10 wks | If gestational age/gender known, write below symbol. Key/legend used to define shading. |
| 11. Termination of pregnancy (TOP) | 18 wks 47,XY,+18 | | Other abbreviations (e.g., TAB, VTOP) not used for sake of consistency. |
| 12. Ectopic pregnancy (ECT) | ECT | | Write ECT below symbol. |

*Source:* Reproduced with permission from Bennett, R. L., et al. (2008). Standardized human pedigree nomenclature: Update and assessment of the recommendations of the National Society of Genetic Counselors. *Journal of Genetic Counseling, 17*, 424–433. DOI 10.1007/s10897-008-9169-9

## Exhibit 3.2 Pedigree Line Definitions

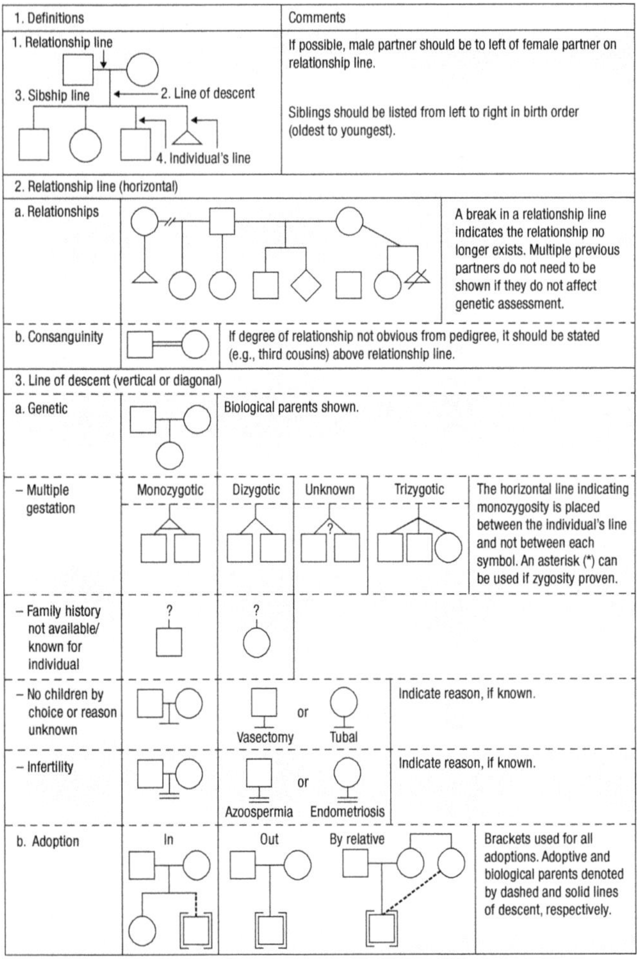


*Source:* Reproduced with permission from Bennett, R. L., et al. (2008). Standardized human pedigree nomenclature: Update and assessment of the recommendations of the National Society of Genetic Counselors. *Journal of Genetic Counseling, 17*, 424–433. DOI 10.1007/s10897-008-9169-9

The goal is to collect a three-generation family health history and to include maternal and paternal relatives. Three generations make it easier to see patterns of inheritance (i.e., dominant, recessive, and

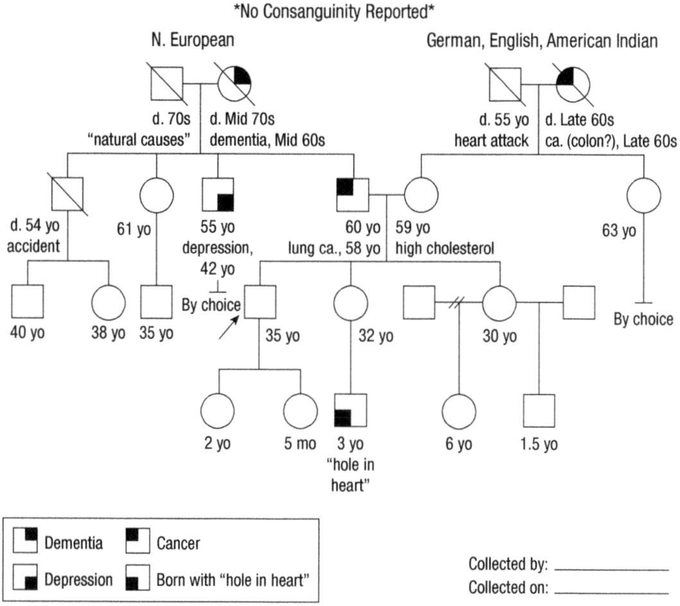


**Figure 3.1** Medical family history: Pedigree.

ca, cancer

X-linked), identify clusters, and recognize genomic red flags. Figure 3.1 contains an example of a three-generation pedigree using standardized symbols.

To orient yourself to the pedigree in Exhibit 3.2, first identify the proband. A proband is the affected individual who brings the family to medical attention or when taking a family history in the primary-care setting, it is your patient. This person is identified by an arrow, and the corresponding symbol is shaded in if they are affected by a disease/disorder you wish to track in the family. The proband acts as the point of reference, and all relationships within the family are designated from the proband's point of view. For example, in the pedigree illustrated in Figure 3.1, the square with an arrow is a 35-year-old male who by history is alive and well (refer to Exhibit 3.1 for the key to pedigree symbols). His first-degree relatives include his two daughters, two sisters, and his parents. His second-degree relatives include his maternal and paternal grandparents (all four are deceased), a maternal aunt, two paternal uncles, one paternal aunt, two nephews, and one niece. He has no third-degree relatives on his mother's side and has three cousins on his father's side of the family. A quick guide to degrees for relationship is provided in Table 3.1.

Table 3.1

Degree of Relationship

| Degree of Relationship | Relative Designation | Percentage of Shared Genes |
| --- | --- | --- |
| First degree | Parents, children, full siblings | 50% (always for parents and children; on average for siblings |
| Second degree | Grandparents, grandchildren, aunts, uncles, nieces, nephews, half siblings | On average 25% |
| Third degree | First cousins | On average 12.5% |

## CREATING THE PEDIGREE

Taking and drawing a medical family history may be comprehensive and involve information on many family members, or it may be targeted to detect a family pattern of a particular condition (e.g., hemophilia) or based on the patient's presenting symptoms (e.g., cancers). The basic approach is the same — collect information about relatives and their partners in one generation and then repeat this moving up and down a generation. Include information on major medical conditions, developmental delays/issues, fertility and maternal health, cause of death, age at disease diagnosis, age at death, and ethnic background. Steps for taking and drawing a family history are summarized in Table 3.2.

**Essential Facts**

Key questions to ask to get the informant(s) ready to create their pedigree with you:

- "Do you have any concerns about conditions or diseases that seem to be running in your family?"
- "Does anyone in your family have a major medical, physical, or mental problem?"
- "Have any adults, children, or babies died? How old were they and what was the cause of death? Have there been any miscarriages or stillbirths? Has anyone had problems becoming pregnant?"

Be systematic in the way in which you go about developing the pedigree. Some clinicians like to draw the family structure first and then

Table 3.2

| Steps for Taking and Drawing a Family History |
|---|
| Ask your informant if they have children and if they are partnered?<br>▪ Do you have children and if so, how many? Have any of your children died, including those who died during pregnancy?<br>▪ Are all your children with the same partner or were any with previous partners?<br>▪ As much as possible draw a siblingship in birth order.<br>Next, ask about each sibling of the informant, their partner(s), and if relevant their children.<br>▪ Remember to ask if any have died as children or during pregnancy.<br>Record details about the parents of your informant.<br>▪ Begin with one of the informant's parents and then repeat the process for the other parent.<br>▪ Record details of each parents' siblings and their children. |
| Collect information on the informant's grandparents, if needed. |
| Now turn to your informant's partner and if relevant collect the same information about their family. |
| Record ancestry and ethnic background on each branch of the family. |
| Develop a key denoting all information relevant to interpreting the pedigree (e.g., define fills and shading and explanations for any abbreviations). |
| If the informant is not the patient (e.g., your patient is a child and a parent is providing the information), denote the historian. |
| Record the date and your name and credentials. |

*Source:* National Genetics and Developmental Centre. (2008). Taking and drawing a family history. https://www.genomicseducation.hee.nhs.uk/

go back and ask for birth/death dates and relevant health and developmental histories. Others collect this information as they draw. Figure 3.1 contains a finished pedigree, which includes the information collected at each step of the process. At first, the pedigree may look cluttered. However, once you understand the symbols and notations, you can see that a pedigree is an effective way to keep a lot of information organized and easily accessible. With family history displayed in this format, you can also easily visualize inheritance patterns or clustering that may make interpretation easier. The family medical history may need to be verified by obtaining medical documentation on other family members.

## Comprehensive Family History

In a general healthcare setting, providers should collect family histories by eliciting general health information about the relatives represented on a patient's pedigree. Examples of conditions to ask about are:

- Major medical concerns
- Chronic medical conditions (for example, something for which medication or therapy is required)
- Hospitalizations or major surgeries
- Birth defects
- Mental retardation, learning disabilities, or developmental delay

### Targeted Family History

A targeted family history is appropriate in a specialized clinical setting or when evaluating a patient for specific concerns. A targeted history includes information about health problems in a patient's relatives that are related to the condition of concern. When evaluating a patient for a certain syndrome, inherited cancer, or heart disease, for example, it would be most beneficial to ask about the presence in other family members of different features associated with that syndrome or condition. A targeted family history would also be appropriate if the general family history reveals a possible inherited condition.

**Essential Facts**

- Taking a family history can take time. Have your patients begin their family history before their visit. These websites provide tools to help your patients collect a family health history:
  - U.S. Surgeon General Family History Initiative: www.hhs.gov/familyhistory
  - Centers for Disease Control and Prevention Family History website: https://www.cdc.gov/genomics/famhistory/index.htm
  - Genetic Alliance: www.geneticalliance.org
  - Heartland Genetics Services Network: https://www.heartlandcollaborative.org/for-families/family-history-tools
- Encourage patients to talk with other family members.
- Be sure to update the information in your patients' pedigrees regularly just like you would for immunization records.

## GENOMIC RED FLAGS

Although charts and lists can be used to assemble family health information, a pedigree is preferred because unlike charts and lists it allows you to quickly visualize patterns (inheritance and familial clustering). When you are taking a targeted family history you often already suspect an inherited condition and patterns of inheritance may be more obvious. Patterns of inheritance include autosomal dominant, autosomal recessive, and X-linked associate with single-gene disorders. These inheritance patterns are presented in detail in Chapter 4. However, sometimes disorders cluster in families without a clear inheritance pattern, or a disorder appears to be manifested in your patient for the first time in a family. In addition to clear inheritance patterns, look for clues and clustering as listed in Table 3.3 that could indicate a strong genetic component and higher risk for other family members.

Table 3.3

**Genomic Red Flags**

| Red Flag | Example |
|---|---|
| Family history of known or suspected inherited condition | Several female first-degree relatives diagnosed with breast cancer |
| Multiple affected family members with same or related disorders | Presence of related disorders in close relatives (e.g., depression, attention deficit disorder, substance use disorder) |
| Earlier age at onset of disease than expected | A 30-year-old male who has a heart attack |
| Developmental delays or mental retardation | A four-year-old male who is not meeting physical developmental milestones—cannot jump or peddle a bike |
| Diagnosis in less-often-affected sex | Breast cancer in a male |
| Multifocal or bilateral occurrence in paired organs | Bilateral hearing loss in a five-year-old female |
| One or more major malformations | A baby born with cleft palate and ventricular septal defect |
| Disease in the absence of risk factors or after preventive measures | A healthy and active 25-year-old female with hypercholesterolemia |
| Abnormalities in growth (growth retardation, asymmetric growth, excessive growth) | Poor growth and delayed signs of puberty in a fifteen-year-old female |
| Recurrent pregnancy losses (3+) | A couple who can conceive a pregnancy but is not able to carry the baby to term |
| Consanguinity (blood relationship of parents) | Mating between cousins |
| Ethnic predisposition to certain genetic disorders | Sickle cell anemia among Black Americans |

## FAMILY HISTORY AND INTERVENTION

While the medical family history is a powerful assessment tool, it can also lead to intervention. Stated previously, information contained in the pedigree forms the basis for shared clinical decision making, which could include referral for clinical or genetic screening/testing and subsequent strategies specific to early intervention or preventative treatments. Additionally, nurses can use the medical family history to explore how their patients assess their own risk and to consequently clarify misconceptions the patient may have about the disorder in question or symptoms they may be experiencing. Creating a shared understanding of what is happening can help patients adjust to prescribed testing and interventions and help with communicating risk to other family members.

## END-OF-CHAPTER QUESTIONS

1. How can the following interfere with the interpretation of a patient's family medical history?
   - Adoption
   - Cultural definitions of family
   - Cultural biases
   - Misattributed paternity
   - Non-traditional families
   - Reliability of information

## VIGNETTE

Risk factors for T2D include being overweight, age, inactivity, high blood pressure, family history, and race/ethnicity. Your patient is 27-year-old Julianna, who is concerned about her risk for developing T2D. Your assessment included the family medical history depicted in the pedigree in Figure 3.2.

It appears that Julianna's relatives with T2D also have one or more T2D risk factors. Factors decreasing risk of a genetic basis include affected family members' having multiple risk factors, some of which are environmental, and affected relatives are older. Factors increasing the risk for genetic basis include a positive family history of T2D in several close relatives, multiple affected family members with same or related disorders, and race. Julianna's risk for developing T2D is higher than the background population risk. However, it is likely that if Julianna stays healthy and avoids lifestyle risk factors, her risk of developing T2D is decreased.

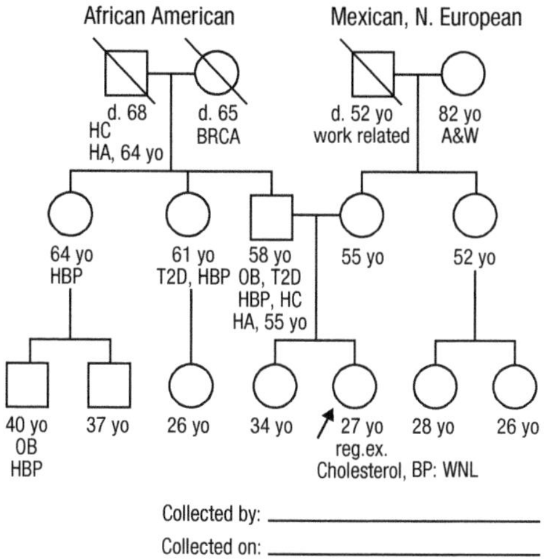


**Figure 3.2** Family medical history: risk for developing type-2 diabetes.

A&W, alive and well; BP, blood pressure; BRCA, breast cancer; HA, heart attack; HBP, high blood pressure; HC, high cholesterol; OB, obese; REG EX, regular exercise; SM, smoker; T2D, type 2 diabetes; WNL, within normal limits

## REFERENCES

Audrain-McGovern, J., Hughes, C., & Patterson, F. (2003). Effecting behavior change: Awareness of family history. *American Journal of Preventive Medicine, 24*(2), 183–189. https://doi.org/10.1016/S0749-3797(02)00592-5

Bennett, R. L., French, K. S., Resta, R. G., & Doyle, D. L. (2008). Standardized human pedigree nomenclature: Update and assessment of the recommendations of the National Society of Genetic Counselors. *Journal of Genetic Counseling, 17*, 424–433. https://doi.org/10.1007/s10897-008-9169-9

National Genetics and Developmental Centre. (2008). *Taking and drawing a family history.* https://www.genomicseducation.hee.nhs.uk/

Scheuner, M. T. (2004). Clinical application of genetic risk assessment strategies for coronary artery disease: genotypes, phenotypes, and family history. *Primary Care: Clinics in Office Practice, 31*, 711–737. https://doi.org/10.1016/j.pop.2004.04.001

Sheehan, E., Bennett, R. L., Harris, M., & Chan-Smutko, G. (2020). Assessing transgender and gender non-conforming pedigree nomenclature in current genetic counselors' practice: The case for geometric inclusivity. *Journal of Genetic Counseling, 29*, 1114–1125. https://doi.org/10.1002/jgc4.1256

Yoon, P. W., Scheuner, M. T., & Khoury, M. J. (2003). Research priorities for evaluating family history in the prevention of common chronic diseases. *American Journal of Preventive Medicine, 4*(2), 128–135. https://doi.org/10.1016/s0749-3797(02)00585-8

# 4

# Patterns of Inheritance

Susan W. Wesmiller and Susan Grayson

*You have learned that building a family pedigree is an essential part of the family history; in fact, many homes proudly display the "Family Tree." In this chapter, we take the next step, using the pedigree constructed in Chapter 3 to determine what we can learn from a pedigree. Even when genetic testing results are not available, the phenotypes of individuals displayed on a pedigree provide essential information from which inheritance patterns can be identified. This chapter provides examples for you to understand the difference between "recessive" and "dominant" alleles and how the work of Mendel is still relevant today. We will also examine other inheritance patterns considered nontraditional, or often non-Mendelian, because they were unknown to Mendel and his peas.*

**In this chapter, you will learn about:**

1. Gregor Mendel, the father of genetics
2. How to use a Punnett square
3. The most common inheritance patterns:
   a. Mendelian autosomal modes of inheritance
   b. X-linked and mitochondrial inheritance
   c. Non-Mendelian modes of inheritance
   d. Multifactorial inheritance

## GREGOR MENDEL

The scientific studies of Gregor Mendel, an Augustinian monk who loved to garden, resulted in what we now call Mendelian patterns of inheritance. Mendel first published his work in 1866, yet it was not noticed until the turn of the century, sadly after he died in 1884. Mendel's work focused on seven different traits of peas. His crossbreeding of pea plants would change the face of genetics. The result of his studies and detailed statistics was that there are distinct hereditary "units," which we now know as genes! He found that when he crossed yellow peas with green peas, there were only yellow peas in the first generation, but in the second generation, there was a 25% probability that there was a green pea! From this observation, he reported that the color yellow was dominant over the color green. Because of his studies of the different traits of peas, we can predict the probability of autosomal dominant and autosomal recessive disorders, described below.

## THE PUNNETT SQUARE

Using the statistics from Mendel's data, Reginald Punnett (Edwards, 2012) invented the Punnett square to provide a method of determining all possible combinations of alleles (genes). Remembering that each parent has two alleles for any one trait, a Punnett square works by placing all possible alleles in a table. For example, Table 4.1 uses Mendel's work to cross two heterozygous peas (one yellow allele and one green allele).

## AUTOSOMAL DOMINANT INHERITANCE

The Punnett square in Table 4.1 demonstrates the dominant trait of yellow peas. Only one variant allele is needed for offspring to inherit the trait or disease in an autosomal inheritance pattern. In the

Table 4.1

**Punnett Square Example**

| | | Paternal Parent | |
|---|---|---|---|
| | | Yellow Dominant | Green Recessive |
| **Maternal Parent** | Yellow Dominant | Y/Y | Y/g |
| | Green Recessive | Y/g | g/g |

Table 4.2

**Huntington Variant**

| | Huntington Variant | Healthy Allele |
|---|---|---|
| Healthy Allele | Huntington/Healthy | Healthy/Healthy |
| Healthy Allele | Huntington/Healthy | Healthy/Healthy |

situation shown with parents who are heterozygous (carry two different alleles) for pea color, the offspring who inherit one yellow allele will have a 75% probability to be yellow. However, in **autosomal dominant** inheritance patterns, only one parent is affected most often.

An example of an autosomal dominant disease is Huntington's disease. Offspring of individuals who carry the Huntington gene pathogenic variant will have a 50% chance of inheriting Huntington's disease. The Punnett Square for an autosomal dominant inheritance pattern with one parent who has been affected by the disease and one who does not carry the condition is shown in Table 4.2.

In the case of autosomal dominant, each offspring has a 50% probability of carrying the Huntington gene. Huntington's disease is an autosomal dominant disorder characterized by adult onset of progressive neurological changes. Important clues to remember about autosomal dominant inheritance patterns when looking at a pedigree are as follows:

- Occurs every generation
- Occurs equally in both biological sexes

## AUTOSOMAL RECESSIVE INHERITANCE

In contrast to autosomal dominant traits, some traits are autosomal recessive. If a person inherits one allele for a recessive trait and one allele for a dominant trait, then the recessive trait will not be displayed. A person must have two recessive alleles to display the recessive phenotype, with one recessive allele from each parent. As shown on the Punnett square for pea colors, only ¼ of the offspring, in this case, would have the recessive trait, or green color.

An example of a recessive trait in a single-gene disorder is cystic fibrosis (CF). For an individual to have CF, they must inherit two recessive variant alleles of the *CFTR* gene. This means that each of their parents must have had at least one recessive allele to pass on to their offspring. Parents who have only one recessive allele, therefore not diagnosed with CF, are called carriers. Carriers do not have the disease or the trait and may not know unless they have genetic testing that they are at risk for passing on the disorder. You will learn more about genetic testing for carriers in a later chapter.

There are certain signs in a pedigree that may be indicative of an autosomal recessive inheritance pattern. Autosomal recessive traits are known to "skip" generations. This means two parents who do not display the trait can have a child with the trait, which does not happen in the case of autosomal dominant traits. However, autosomal recessive traits appear with equal frequency across sexes, like autosomal dominant traits.

**Essential Facts**

If a parent with blue eyes and a parent with brown eyes have a child with blue eyes, the blue eyes actually come from the parent with brown eyes! Since blue eyes are recessive and brown eyes are dominant, the blue-eyed parent must have two blue alleles and would pass on a blue allele no matter what. However, for the child to have blue eyes, they must also have two blue alleles, meaning one came from their brown-eyed parent. The brown-eyed parent can have one brown allele and one blue allele. Even two brown-eyed parents can have a blue-eyed child if they each carry a blue allele!

## X-LINKED

While both autosomal dominant and autosomal recessive traits appear with equal frequency across the sexes, X-linked traits do not follow this pattern. Individuals that are genetically female have two X-chromosomes, meaning they receive two alleles for every gene on the X-chromosome. On the other hand, Males only have one X-chromosome as well as one Y-chromosome. This means that if a male has a particular allele for an X-linked gene, he will not have another allele for that gene from the Y-chromosome, which is called hemizygosity. If a male is hemizygous for an X-linked recessive trait, they will not have another allele for that trait, meaning the trait will be expressed. However, suppose a female inherits one allele for an X-linked recessive trait. In that case, there will also be an allele on the other X-chromosome, causing the female to be heterozygous, and the recessive trait will not be expressed. Females need two copies of an X-linked recessive allele for the recessive trait to be expressed, while males only need one copy. This is why X-linked recessive traits

Table 4.3

Gender Patterns

| | $X_1$ | $X_2$ |
|---|---|---|
| X | $X, X_1$ | $X, X_2$ |
| Y | $X_1, Y$ | $X_2, Y$ |

are more frequently observed in males, and pedigrees of X-linked traits show sex-linked patterns of inheritance. A Punnett square for X-linked disorders is very different, as shown here. The maternal X's are labeled as $X_1$ and $X_2$, with *$X_2$ the affected allele*. Because the female offspring here do not carry two affected X's, they will not inherit the phenotype. Males have a 50% probability of inheriting the X-linked disorder (Table 4.3).

Some specific patterns can be observed with X-linked recessive traits, an example of which is red-green colorblindness. If a male has red-green colorblindness, he will pass on the colorblind allele to his female offspring because only the X-chromosome he has to give has the colorblind allele. However, a male with red-green colorblindness cannot pass the allele on to any of his male offspring, because they have all received a Y-chromosome from him instead of the X-chromosome with the colorblind allele. This is often referred to as male-to-male transmission, which does not occur with X-linked traits. On the other hand, a female with red-green colorblindness will pass the trait on to all her male offspring since both of her X-chromosomes that she might pass on to him have the colorblind allele. However, suppose she mates with a male without colorblindness. In that case, their female offspring will be carriers for colorblindness but not display the trait, because they received an X-chromosome without the allele for colorblindness from their father.

## MITOCHONDRIAL

While the genes and alleles that have been referred to so far have been from genetic material in the nucleus of the cell, some traits can be passed on through a smaller amount of genetic material in the cellular mitochondria. What is unique about this type of inheritance is that offspring only receive mitochondria from their female parent. This means that mitochondrial traits are passed on from a female parent to all of her offspring. However, males with the trait will not pass on the trait to their offspring.

Since mitochondria are responsible for cellular metabolism, many disorders with mitochondrial inheritance patterns are related to metabolic dysfunctions. An example of a mitochondrial inherited disorder is Leigh syndrome, a metabolic disorder that affects the central nervous system.

The process of mitochondrial inheritance can be complicated by the concept of heteroplasmy. This occurs when there is more than one type of mitochondrial DNA in a cell. The severity of some conditions caused by variations in mitochondrial DNA can be affected by the proportion of mitochondria in the cells with the DNA variant. Additionally, there is no guarantee that the ratio of mitochondria with the DNA variant will remain constant through reproduction, allowing the severity of these conditions to change across generations.

## CHARACTERISTICS OF NON-TRADITIONAL INHERITANCE PATTERNS

### Variable Expressivity

Even among people with the same genetic condition, different signs and symptoms of the condition may be expressed. This is referred to as **variable** expressivity. Signs and symptoms of genetic conditions can vary in severity or in how they are expressed. An example of a disease with variable expressivity is Marfan syndrome. All individuals with Marfan syndrome (an autosomal dominant condition) will have a mutation in the *FBN1* gene. However, while some individuals with Marfan syndrome may present only with abnormally long and thin limbs, others may have heart conditions, vision problems, or spinal abnormalities.

## PENETRANCE

Penetrance is related to the proportion of individuals with a genotype who actually display the associated trait. For example, if only 70% of a population with an allele for a trait actually demonstrates that trait, the allele is said to have 70% penetrance (Klug et al., 2019). In any case, where the penetrance is less than 100%, meaning there are individuals who have the genotype but do not display the trait, the trait is said to have incomplete penetrance. An example of an allele with incomplete penetrance is the *BRCA1* gene, a gene in which a mutation can lead to familial breast cancer. An estimated 57% of individuals with a mutation in the *BRCA1* gene will develop breast cancer (Chen & Parmigiani, 2007), giving a variant *BRCA1* allele 57% penetrance.

While variable expressivity and incomplete penetrance are related concepts, there are key differences. While variable expressivity is pertaining to individual differences in the way a trait is expressed, penetrance can be thought of as a statistical construct expressing the likelihood that an individual with a specific allele will express the trait at all. To illustrate, we can examine polydactyly, a condition with variable expressivity and incomplete penetrance. Polydactyly is a genetic condition where individuals have extra digits. However, some individuals who have inherited an allele for polydactyly will not have any extra digits, indicating incomplete penetrance. Among the individuals with the allele who do have extra digits, the location, size, or number of extra digits may vary. One individual may have a small stub for an extra toe, while another might have a complete extra finger. These differences demonstrate variable expressivity.

## INCOMPLETE DOMINANCE

Incomplete dominance occurs when an individual who is heterozygous does not entirely display the dominant trait but instead expresses an intermediate phenotype. Instead of one allele being completely dominant over another, the two alleles "compromise" on the phenotype. An easy-to-picture example of this can be found in flowers. The allele for a red flower has incomplete dominance over the allele for a white flower, causing plants with one red allele and one white allele to have pink flowers.

## CO-DOMINANCE

In the case of co-dominance, there are multiple alleles for a trait that can be expressed simultaneously without one dominant allele inhibiting the expression of another dominant allele. An example of co-dominance can be seen in human blood types. If a person has an allele for an A blood type and an allele for a B blood type, their blood type will be AB, with neither allele preventing the expression of the other. However, both A and B are dominant over O-type blood. Since O-type blood is recessive, an individual with that blood type must carry both O alleles.

Co-dominance is different from incomplete dominance in that co-dominant alleles are both fully expressed in an individual, but alleles with incomplete dominance are only partially expressed, leading to an intermediate expression of the phenotype or the pink flowers.

**Essential Facts**

Parents have four children representing all the possible phenotypes for blood type. You know that one parent must carry an O allele and a B allele, and the other parent then must carry an O allele and an A allele. The result would be the ***phenotypes*** for four blood types: A, B, AB, O. The ***genotypes*** for the parents would be A-O, B-O, A-B, and O-O.

## MULTIFACTORIAL INHERITANCE

Multifactorial traits are the result of both polygenic and environmental influences. A good example is coronary artery disease. Hundreds of genetic variants have been associated with cardiovascular disorders, most adding a small part to the overall genetic risk (Gladding et al., 2020). The collective contribution by these genetic variants working together increases the risk for coronary artery disease. In addition to this overall genetic risk, it is well known that obesity, lack of exercise, and increased stress also contribute to coronary artery disease, resulting in multifactorial genetic and environmental contributing factors. Before the availability of genome-wide association studies (GWAS) that were made possible after completing the Human Genome Project (described in an earlier chapter), it was challenging to determine diseases caused by multiple genes (Jorde, Carey & Bamshad, 2021). GWAS studies and reliance on statistical analysis now provide a better understanding of the multiple variables and the overall genetic risk leading to multifactorial inheritance.

## CONCLUSION

This chapter discussed the most common inheritance patterns: autosomal dominant, autosomal recessive, X-linked, mitochondrial, and multifactorial. It is not always easy to determine the exact pattern from a pedigree, but recognizing the most common types of inheritance patterns in the situations presented will help you understand individuals at risk.

## REFERENCES

Chen, S., & Parmigiani, G. (2007). Meta-analysis of BRCA1 and BRCA2 penetrance. *Journal of Clinical Oncology: Official Journal of the American*

*Society of Clinical Oncology, 25*(11), 1329–1333. https://doi.org/10.1200/JCO.2006.09.1066

Edwards, A. (2012). Reginald Crundall Punnett: First Arthur Balfour professor of genetics, Cambridge, 1912. *Genetics, 192*, 3–13.

Gladding, P., Legget, M., Fatkin, D., Larsen, P., & Doughty, R. (2020). Polygenic risk scores in coronary artery disease and atrial fibrillation. *Heart, Lung and Circulation, 29*, 634–640.

Jorde, L., Carey, J., & Bamshad, M. (2021). *Medical genetics* (6th ed.). Elsevier.

Klug, W., Cummings, M., Spencer, C., Palladino, M., & Killian, D. (2019). *Concepts of genetics* (12th ed.). Pearson Education, Inc.

# 5

# Cancer Genetics: When a Good Cell Behaves Badly

Deborah Tamura

*Approximately 1,898,160 new cases of cancer will be diagnosed in the United States in 2021, and an estimated 608,570 people will die from it. Despite advances in screening, diagnosis, and treatment, cancer continues to be the second leading cause of death in the United States (https://seer.cancer.gov/statfacts/html/all.html and www.cc.gov).*

*Cancer is a genetic disease at the molecular level. Essentially, all cancers arise from a normal cell that has accumulated a series of mutations (alterations in the DNA), resulting in a dysregulated growth pattern. In this chapter you will learn about the basic mechanisms of normal cell growth and division. You will learn how chromosome and DNA damage can occur. You will appreciate how the cell maintains normal DNA integrity through various repair processes that prevent the accumulation of DNA damage, which otherwise would result in mutations. When the damage is not corrected, the immune system performs an important check on abnormal cells, serving as the final step in the prevention of cancer development. You will also learn about inherited genetic conditions, including those in immune function and DNA repair pathways, that can lead to an increased risk of cancer development.*

*DNA-damaging agents in the environment, or carcinogens, also play a role in cancer development. Carcinogens (cancer-causing agents) are ubiquitous in the environment and include some commonly encountered substances, like cigarette smoke, and it is often necessary for repeated carcinogen exposures before cancer results. Cancer clusters may be seen in employees who work in mining, petrochemical plants, and other businesses associated with high carcinogen exposure. Links to several carcinogen databases are included in this chapter.*

*A more thorough understanding of cancer genetics has led to the development of better therapeutic agents. As research continues into the genetic abnormalities of tumors, advances in newer, more effective treatments will result in better outcomes for cancer patients.*

**In this chapter, you will learn:**

1. To describe the basic changes in DNA that lead to the development of cancer
2. To list methods DNA uses to repair damage
3. To identify common environmental carcinogens
4. To recognize signs of hereditary cancer risk in a family health history
5. To explain the basic mechanism of targeted chemotherapy agents and immunotherapy

## HOW CANCER OCCURS: MISTAKES HAPPEN

The cell cycle is the process a cell undergoes during normal function, growth, and division. It is a series of tightly regulated steps during which the cell performs normal metabolic functions, grows, synthesizes DNA, and finally doubles chromosomes and other cellular material to make two exact copies. In this section, we will be discussing the cell cycle events of actively dividing somatic cells (Tessema et al., 2004). Table 5.1 lists the steps of the cell cycle and describes the properties of each step.

Somatic cells that have fully differentiated, such as smooth muscle cells, nerves, and heart and retina cells, rarely divide and remain in an interphase step of the cell cycle and perform their prescribed metabolic functions. Neurons may stay in a state of interphase for decades. However, rapidly dividing cells can complete all the steps of the cell cycle very quickly. For example, cells in the intestine or cornea of the eye can complete the cell cycle in 24 hours (Mao et al., 2012;

Table 5.1

**Cell Cycle**

| Stages of Cell Cycle | Properties of Cell Cycle Behavior |
|---|---|
| G1 – Gap1 | Cell is performing normal programmed activity; period of cell growth if this is a cell that actively divides. |
| S – Synthesis | Cell copies or synthesizes DNA; copying errors may occur, leading to DNA mutations. |
| G2 – Gap 2 | Checking of DNA for copy errors occurs through the activity of DNA repair enzymes; cell prepares to divide. |
| Mitosis | Division of the doubled DNA strands. Includes prophase, anaphase, metaphase, and telophase; errors during mitosis can result in abnormal chromosome numbers, deletions, or translocations of part or all of a chromosome. |
| Cytokinesis | Splitting of cytoplasm and cellular organelles between the two daughter cells following mitosis of the chromosomes in the nucleus. |
| G0 | Cell is in a quiescent phase; may be an extended G1 phase or a stage occurring out of the cell cycle. |
| Interphase | Any cell that is in G1, S, or G2—a nondividing cell |

Tessema et al., 2004). Cells must divide to cause cancer, and cancers occur more often in rapidly dividing cells, such as epithelial cells in the cervix and lung (Rogalla & Contag, 2015).

## CHROMOSOME ABNORMALITIES IN CANCER CELLS

Given the multitude of DNA that is synthesized, copied, and segregated, the cell cycle is a remarkably accurate process. Each somatic cell contains approximately 3.2 billion base pairs of DNA, and these base pairs must be faithfully copied for normal function of the daughter cells (Nachman & Crowell, 2000). Although the replication of DNA and segregation of the 23 pairs of chromosomes is extremely precise, errors do happen. Chromosome missegregation can result in daughter cells with extra or missing chromosomes or only parts of a chromosome. A section of a chromosome may break and reattach to another chromosome (translocation) or be "broken off" and lost (chromosome deletion). Cells with abnormal numbers of chromosomes or abnormal configurations of chromosomes are termed aneuploid cells. Cancer cells often exhibit aneuploidy, and approximately 90% of cancer cells have either lost or gained a chromosome. Over 80%

Table 5.2

**Aneuploidy in Common Cancer Cells**

| Cancer Type | Commonly Seen Chromosome Abnormalities |
|---|---|
| Glioblastoma | Gain of chromosome 7, loss of chromosome 10; gain of bottom arm of chromosome 19, loss of top arm of chromosome 1 |
| Lung cancer – squamous cell | Gain of bottom arm of chromosome 3, loss of top arm of chromosome 3 |
| Lung cancer – adenocarcinoma | Gain of bottom arm of chromosome 1; gain of top arm of chromosome 7 |
| Gastrointestinal cancers | Gain of bottom arms of chromosomes 3 and 8; gain of chromosome 13 |
| Hematologic malignancies and myelodysplastic syndromes | Loss of bottom arm of chromosome 20; loss of bottom arm of chromosome 5 |
| Lymphoma neoplasms | Loss of section of top arm of chromosome 1; loss or gain of bottom arm of chromosome 11 |
| Prostate cancer | Gain of part of top arm of chromosome 16; gain or loss in part of bottom arm of chromosome 8 |

*Source:* From Kou, F., Wu, L., Ren, X., & Yang, L. (2020). Chromosome abnormalities: New insights into their clinical significance in cancer. *Molecular Therapy – Oncolytics, 17*, 562–570. https://doi.org/10.1016/j.omto.2020.05.010

of chromosomes in cancer cells have deleted and/or amplified (extra copies of) chromosome arms (Kou et al., 2020). Chromothripsis is a particularly devastating chromosomal event for a cell. This is a massive genomic rearrangement occurring in a single event and is usually isolated or localized to specific chromosome regions. This can be an initiating event for cancer development (Table 5.2) (Harbers et al., 2021).

In addition to containing extra or missing chromosomes or chromosome segments, cancer cells have mutations in individual genes important for cell division. These genes are critical to maintaining a normal balance in cell growth. A "protooncogene" is a gene that is important to cell proliferation, growth, and differentiation. It also functions in control of the cell cycle and in halting apoptosis (cell death). When a protooncogene is mutated, termed an oncogene, it contributes to an abnormal increase in cell growth. Tumor-suppressor genes are genes that act to stop or slow cell division. They can arrest the cell cycle from progressing through the gap phases to mitosis. This arrest allows mistakes to be corrected by DNA damage-repair mechanisms before the cell divides. Tumor-suppressor genes can also function by inducing apoptosis (cell death) when the cell contains significant damage. Together the two types of genes act like an accelerator and brake in a car. The oncogenes act as an accelerator to "speed up" the cell growth and division; the tumor-suppressor genes act as the brake to "slow down" or stop cell division and proliferation. It is this balance between the actions of tumor-suppressor genes and protooncogenes that keep a cell dividing only when signaled to do so. When this balance is disrupted, the process of malignant transformation or carcinogenesis can occur (Kou et al., 2020; Stanbridge, 1990).

## CARCINOGENESIS

Carcinogenesis is the process by which a normal cell accumulates sufficient DNA damage to be transformed into a cancer cell. DNA damage itself is not a mutation. However, mutations (a change in the normal sequence of DNA) resulting in cancer are derived from DNA damage. Table 5.3 lists the steps of carcinogenesis.

Table 5.3

**Steps in Carcinogenesis**

| Initiation | Promotion | Transformation/ Malignant Conversion | Tumor Progression |
|---|---|---|---|
| Cancer begins with mutations in genes controlling growth pathways or from chromosome abnormalities. However, at this phase the cell continues to grow normally. | The cell accumulates additional mutations that promote more rapid cell division. The cell may be dividing more rapidly but continues to respond to signaling. | Accumulation of multiple gene mutations and chromosome abnormalities over time. Significantly enhanced growth and survival of cell. Cell is a precancer. | Cell has accumulated substantial numbers of mutations and is no longer responding to cellular growth-control signaling. Can eventually metastasize. Cell has become malignant. |
| Cell is visibly normal in pathology specimens. | | Cell is visibly abnormal in pathology specimens. | Cell appears very abnormal and is rapidly dividing. Mitotic figures can be seen in pathology specimens. |

Cancer initiation begins when damaged DNA results in mutations in genes important for cell division. It is necessary for there to be an accumulation of DNA damage and mutations over a period of time for a cell to progress from a normal cell to a cancer cell. The DNA damage can occur either by an external source (exogenous damage) or by endogenous sources, such as a mistake in DNA synthesis during the cell cycle. It is estimated that when a cell divides, it accumulates approximately 175 mutations per cell division (Nachman & Crowell, 2000). Most of these mutations are of little or no consequence to cellular function; however, if a mutation(s) occurs in protooncogenes, tumor-suppressor genes, or genes important for DNA repair, or if an aneuploidy event occurs, they can be initiating events for cancer.

As a cell experiences multiple events of DNA damage, such as aneuploidy and gene mutations, it may continue to progress to malignant transformation. This process was first clearly delineated in colon cancer. Fearon and Vogelstein (1990) described the loss and gain of functions for tumor suppressor and protooncogenes in precancerous and cancerous colonic epithelial cells. They identified each pathological abnormality in the progression from a normal colon epithelial cell through various stages of adenomas to colon cancer. They then linked each stage of pathologic change with specific acquired genetic abnormalities.

Important DNA abnormalities have also been identified in other cancers, such as chronic myelogenous leukemia. An aneuploidy event (translocation) occurs between chromosomes 9 and 22 (the Philadelphia chromosome), resulting in the gain of function of a protooncogene, tyrosine kinase. This gain of function results in an alteration of gene function, leading eventually to the overproduction of abnormal immature myeloid cells and the development of chronic myelogenous leukemia (Kou et al., 2020).

Tumor-suppressor genes act to stop or slow down the process of carcinogenesis. The powerful tumor-suppressor gene *TP53* initiates the apoptosis or cell-death cascade when a cell is very abnormal or has experienced substantial damage. The *TP53* gene is an extremely important tumor-suppressor gene and is either nonfunctioning, mutated, or lost in many cancer tumors. Another tumor -suppressor gene, *RB1*, acts to control cell division by slowing down the expression of growth-activating factors (signaling) in the cell. This tumor-suppressor gene is important in regulating cell growth in the retina and many other tissues. Tumor-suppressor genes usually sustain inactivating mutations during the DNA synthesis step of the cell cycle. Tumor-suppressor genes can also be deleted when chromosomes or parts of chromosomes are lost during mitosis. Mutations in tumor-suppressor genes result in a decreased capacity to respond to abnormal cell growth, leading to increased proliferation of progressively atypical cells. Without normally functioning tumor-suppressor genes, there are few blocks on the continued growth of abnormal cells, possibly leading to the development of cancer. A cancer tumor contains many cells containing a wide array of mutations. Table 5.4 is a small list of protooncogenes and tumor-suppressor genes with their functions and related cancers (Kou et al., 2020).

Table 5.4

**Representative List of Protooncogenes and Tumor-Suppressor Genes With Their Functions and Cancer Type**

| Gene | Function | Cancer |
| --- | --- | --- |
| *AKT2* Oncogene | Encodes for a protein kinase – "energizes" cell | Ovarian cancer |
| *MYC (c-MYC)* Oncogene | Promotes cell proliferation and DNA synthesis | Leukemia, breast, stomach, lung, and other cancers |
| *EGFR* Oncogene | Triggers cell growth by interacting with tyrosine kinase | Squamous cell carcinoma, glioblastoma, lung cancer |
| *ERBB2* Oncogene | Interacts with tyrosine kinase | Breast cancer, salivary gland cancer, ovarian cancer |
| *HRAS, KRAS, NRAS* Oncogenes | Act in signal transduction (passing information) from cell surface to interior | Bladder, lung, ovarian, and breast cancers |
| *APC* Tumor-Suppressor Gene | Slows transcription and homeostasis of some genes | Colon cancer |
| *BRCA1* and *2* Tumor-Suppressor Gene | Functions in DNA damage repair | Breast and ovarian cancers |
| *CDKN2A* Tumor-Suppressor Gene | Regulates cell cycle passage from G1 into S | Melanoma |
| *TP53* Tumor-Suppressor Gene | Functions in cell cycle; arrests cell cycle in G1 phase; initiates apoptosis | Bladder, breast, colorectal, liver, lung, prostate, and many other cancers |
| *VHL* Tumor-Suppressor Gene | Cell cycle regulation; may increase activity of *P53* | Renal cancer |

### Chromosome Abnormalities: New Insights Into Their Clinical Significance in Cancer

In conclusion, the process of carcinogenesis occurs when there is an accumulation of multiple genetic abnormalities in a cell, leading to dysregulated cellular growth. Cancer cells often demonstrate profound chromosome abnormalities. The abnormalities in chromosomes can result in the upregulation of protooncogenes by moving them to new locations or by adding additional copies of protooncogenes. These chromosome abnormalities also result in the loss of tumor-suppressor genes. The tumor-suppressor genes are lost in cancer cells by the deletion of chromosome arms or through the loss of whole chromosomes (Kou et al., 2020).

## JUST HOW MANY WAYS CAN YOU DAMAGE DNA?

There are many ways to damage DNA, such as chromosome abnormalities and gene mutations that place a cell on the path to carcinogenesis. Mutations in certain genes are more critical to the process of carcinogenesis, providing a cell with a growth and survival advantage. Driver mutations are mutations in those genes that initiate and continue the progress of carcinogenesis and provide a survival advantage to the cancer cell. However, not all gene mutations are critical to this process, and mutations in genes less critical or not important to carcinogenesis are termed passenger mutations.

There are two basic mechanisms through which DNA damage occurs; the first is endogenous damage. Endogenous damage occurs from replication errors in DNA synthesis during the cell cycle or from the damaging effects of the normal biochemical process associated with cellular metabolism, such as oxidative damage. Endogenous DNA damage can result in missing DNA bases and incorrectly added or deleted bases. It can also cause additions or deletions of large stretches of DNA. This damage is common and occurs at $10^{-6}$ to $10^{-8}$ mutations per cell division. Both processes, replication errors and cellular metabolism, are naturally occurring events in a cell. Replication errors and damage from cellular metabolism can lead to cancer and also result in normal aging (Chatterjee & Walker, 2017; Rizza et al., 2021). Although the development of cancer is often largely attributed to exogenous damage, endogenous DNA damage is a constant threat to genomic integrity and for cancer development (Chatterjee & Walker, 2017; Cheung-Ong et al., 2013).

The second DNA-damaging process is exogenous DNA damage. Exogenous DNA damage occurs because of external substances such as ionizing radiation (IR), ultraviolet radiation (UVR), and chemical agents. Oncology has taken advantage of the DNA-damaging properties of IR and certain chemicals to treat cancer. As examples, damage from IR often causes severe chromosome abnormalities and DNA damage in cancer cells (and to a lesser extent in normal cells in the treatment field), leading to the death of cancer cells. The metabolism of the anthracycline family of chemotherapy drugs (such as doxorubicin and daunomycin) results in large amounts of a form of oxygen radical (superoxide $O_2^-$), which is severely DNA damaging, leading to the death of cancer cells (Ravi & Das, 2004).

The gene mutations caused by both endogenous and exogenous damage include missense mutations (a mutation resulting from a single base pair substitution, which alters the genetic code), nonsense mutations (a mutation that changes an amino acid to a STOP signal in the DNA), and base deletions or insertions (bases that are either left out or added in the DNA). These mutations can result in the loss of function of tumor-suppressor genes or in the upregulation of protooncogenes.

Epigenetic modifications are a different type of gene modification that can result in the down regulation of tumor suppressor and upregulation of oncogenes. Although not directly affecting the DNA or protein sequence of a gene, epigenetic modifications can "turn off" the ability of the gene to be expressed or drive the expression of abnormal or mutated genes. Methylation is the most thoroughly understood epigenetic modification. Methylation occurs when a methyl group is added to a specific place in a gene, termed methylation marks. Methylation is important for many normal cellular processes and in fetal development. However, abnormal methylation can lead to cancer development. Since methylation is not a permanent change in the DNA structure of a gene, the methylation marks can be removed, returning a gene to normal function. This reversable characteristic of methylation is an active area of chemotherapy development (Zhou et al., 2021).

A very dire type of DNA damage occurs when one or both strands of DNA (coding strand and noncoding strands) are broken, termed **strand breaks.** This often leads to serious cellular consequences, including cell death. DNA strand breaks can also result in major DNA rearrangements, such as whole-gene translocations or deletions. Deletions can result in the loss of function of a gene, whereas translocations can result in a gain of function of a gene or the production of a new protein, glycoproteins, glycolipids, or carbohydrates. Often these new cell products act as tumor antigens. Mutations in genes that code for proteins or regulate other genes in the cell are important to progression in carcinogenesis (Aparicio et al., 2014).

## METASTASIS: LEAVING HOME

A cancer tumor evolves due to accumulated mutations in cells. The initial "cancer cell" divides, leading to more cancer cells that are often more abnormal. Eventually a group of cells has accumulated so many mutations, it has the ability to leave the original tumor site, a process termed metastasis. Metastasis is the process by which a cancer cell breaks away from the original tumor and spreads to nearby tissues or more distant sites in the body. Over 90% of cancer deaths are caused by metastasis of malignant cells from the initial tumor. Cancer cells accomplish metastasis by aggressive growth into adjacent normal tissue, invading walls of nearby lymph nodes or blood vessels and migrating through the lymphatic system and bloodstream to settle in other parts of the body. They can stop in small blood vessels at a new location (often far away from the original cancer), invade through the wall of the blood vessel, and move into the surrounding tissue. Metastases often pathologically resemble the tissue of origin. For example, the lung metastases from breast cancer resemble breast tissue, rather than lung tissue. Investigations have found that the process of metastasis occurs over several years after the initial tumor has been identified. The clinical course of metastasis is very different between types of cancers and even within one type of tumor. Research has found that multiple driver mutations in tumor cells and other mutations allow the metastasizing cells to survive until they reach a suitable site. Recent research has also found that specific tissue sites, termed metastatic niches, provide a receptive location for the implantation of tumor cells. Metastatic niches may be "prepared" to receive the disseminated cells years before the metastatic tumors are detectable (Peitzsch et al., 2017).

A relatively new finding in cancer research has been the identification of cancer stem cells within a tumor. Cancer stem cells are a group of tumor cells that can drive tumor initiation and/or can cause tumor relapses. Cancer stem cells are usually treatment resistant and can activate multiple pathways within a tumor to trigger tumor relapse and metastasis (Walcher et al., 2020). Much cancer research is being done to determine which of the many mutations in a cancer are driver or passenger mutations and what mutations characterize a cancer stem cell. Driver mutations in a malignant tumor can result in the local recurrence of a tumor or distant metastasis. In addition, certain types of driver mutations are currently being targeted for new chemotherapeutic drug development.

## Essential Facts

- The cell cycle is a closely controlled series of steps a cell undergoes to perform metabolic functions, grow, and divide.
- Cancer is a genetic disease at the molecular level. It is characterized by the accumulation of DNA damage, resulting in chromosome and gene mutations in cells.
- Carcinogenesis is the process by which a normal cell accumulates sufficient damage and mutations of growth-regulating genes to permit cancer to develop.
- Specific genes termed oncogenes and tumor-suppressor genes function together to regulate cell division. When oncogenes and tumor-suppressor genes accumulate mutations and are no longer functioning properly, unregulated cell growth and cancer can result.
- Driver mutations occur in genes important for the regulation of cell growth and survival. Mutated driver genes are often proto-oncogenes. Mutations in genes considered to be driver genes may be some of the initiating steps in carcinogenesis. Mutations in passenger genes do not appear to significantly affect cell function.
- Metastasis is the process by which malignant cells leave the primary tumor either by direct extension into the local tumor environment or through entry into the circulatory system and/or lymphatic system. Approximately 90% of cancer deaths are due to metastatic disease.

## Maintaining DNA Integrity: Fixing the Mistakes

When DNA is damaged in dividing cells, the damaged DNA lesions stimulate checkpoint pathways, activating specific DNA damage response mechanisms. The DNA damage response mechanisms often arrest the cell cycle until the damage is repaired (Figure 5.1). Once the cell has repaired the damage, the arrested cell resumes cell-cycle progression. If a cell has sustained severe damage that cannot be repaired, it undergoes apoptosis (cell death) or permanent cell-cycle arrest; the cell will no longer be capable of division (Branzei & Foiani, 2008).

The DNA damage response is the process by which DNA damage is identified and repaired. There are multiple DNA damage repair mechanisms (pathways) protecting the integrity of a cell's DNA (Figure 5.1). The pathways either remove the damage, help the cell tolerate damage by eliciting senescence (stay in a permanent

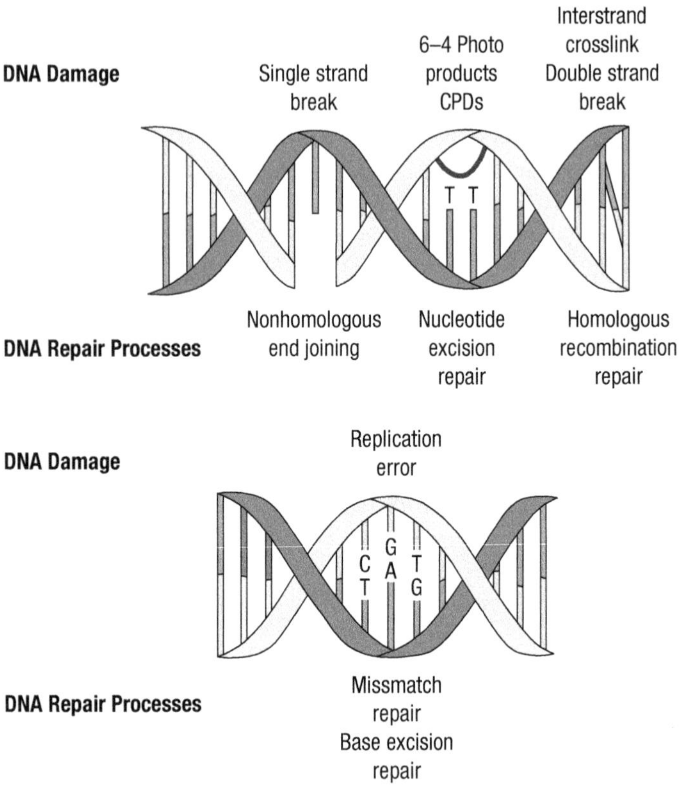


**Figure 5.1** DNA damage and repair.

nonreplicative state), bypass the damage or eliminate a seriously damaged or malfunctioning cell through various cell-death pathways such as apoptosis. These repair mechanisms are important in preventing the overall outcome of DNA damage's leading to mutations and are critical to the prevention of cancer (Ciccia & Elledge, 2010; DiGiovanna & Kraemer, 2012; Mao et al., 2012).

The DNA damage response has evolved over eons to correct most forms of DNA damage encountered by the cell. Table 5.5 lists the major DNA repair pathways, the types of DNA damage that are repaired, and some of the cancers associated when DNA damage is not properly repaired through a pathway. The damage may be caused by endogenous factors, such as replication errors and metabolic stress, or by exogenous agents, including mutagenic and carcinogenic factors. These repair pathways are active in all tissues in the body depending on the type of DNA damage that has occurred.

Table 5.5

**DNA Repair Pathways Recognize and Repair Multiple Forms of DNA Damage**

| DNA Repair Pathway | DNA Damage Repaired | Tissues | Cancers |
|---|---|---|---|
| BER | Small lesions (often single-base abnormalities) caused by replication errors and oxidative and other biochemical damage | Most important DNA repair system; critical to all cells | Cancers of the GI tract, lung cancer, breast cancer |
| NER | Bulky DNA-distorting lesions often caused by ultraviolet radiation or oxidative damage | Important for repair in sun-exposed tissues; skin, oral mucosa, sun-exposed ocular tissues. Oxidative damage in the nervous system | Squamous cell, basal cell carcinomas, melanoma in the skin and eye tissues, papillary thyroid cancer. and several types of CNS tumors |
| Homologous End Joining and NHEJ | Double-strand DNA breaks: both coding and noncoding strands are broken. Double-strand breaks are the most lethal of the forms of DNA damage. | Any tissues exposed to ionizing radiation or chemicals such as alkylating agents Bone marrow, central nervous system tissues often affected | Breast cancer, leukemia, ovarian cancer, lung cancer |
| Single-Strand Break Repair | Single-strand breaks are often caused by oxidative damage and cause the collapse of DNA replication. | Central nervous system and other tissue susceptible to oxidative damage | Breast cancer, leukemia Neurodegenerative conditions |

(continued)

Table 5.5

**DNA Repair Pathways Recognize and Repair Multiple Forms of DNA Damage (*continued*)**

| DNA Repair Pathway | DNA Damage Repaired | Tissues | Cancers |
|---|---|---|---|
| Intrastrand or Interstrand Cross-Link Repair | DNA cross-linking damage occurs when DNA-damaging agents connect two pieces of DNA from the same strand (intrastrand crosslink) or from opposite strands (ICL). Crosslinking damage interrupts essential processes in the cell, including replication and transcription. | Important repair pathway for bone marrow, esophageal tissue, cervix, oral mucosa | Leukemia, bone marrow failure syndromes, head and neck squamous cell carcinoma. Any tissue exposed to exogenous crosslinking agents, including cancer chemotherapy |
| Mismatch Repair | Repairs errors in DNA after cells divide; ensures fidelity of DNA sequences | Important for repair in intestinal epithelium, pancreatic system, and urinary tract | Colon, pancreatic, stomach, endometrial, and urinary tract cancers |
| Bypass Repair | DNA TLS. Translesion polymerases bypass DNA-damage lesions during DNA replication | Skin, lung | Melanoma, lung cancer |

BER, base excision repair; ICL, interstrand crosslink; NER, nucleotide excision repair; NHEJ, non-homologous end joining; TLS, translesion synthesis

*Source*: From Aparicio, T., Baer, R., & Gautier, J. (2014). DNA double-strand break repair pathway choice and cancer. *DNA Repair*, *19*, 169–175. https://doi.org/10.1016/j.dnarep.2014.03.014; DiGiovanna, J. J., & Kraemer, K. H. (2012). Shining a light on xeroderma pigmentosum. *Journal of Investigative Dermatology*, *132*(3 Pt 2), 785–796. https://doi.org/10.1038/jid.2011.426; Hsieh, P., & Yamane, K. (2008). DNA mismatch repair: Molecular mechanism, cancer, and ageing. *Mechanisms of Ageing and Development*, *129*(7–8), 391–407. https://doi.org/10.1016/j.mad.2008.02.012; Huang, Y., & Li, L. (2013). DNA crosslinking damage and cancer – A tale of friend and foe. *Translational Cancer Research*, *2*(3), 144–154. https://doi.org/10.3978/j.issn.2218-676X.2013.03.01; Wallace, S. S., Murphy, D. L., & Sweasy, J. B. (2012). Base excision repair and cancer. *Cancer Letters*, *327*(1–2), 73–89. https://doi.org/10.1016/j.canlet.2011.12.038.

All DNA repair pathways follow the same basic steps: first, the damage must be identified; second, the damage must be accessed; third, the damage must undergo specific repair steps and be removed from the DNA; in the last step, the ends of the repaired strand or strands must be joined. In some cases, the cell does not repair the damage and translesion synthesis polymerases bypass the DNA damage, permitting the cell cycle to continue. It is beyond the scope of this chapter to discuss each DNA damage pathway separately; however, we will cover the nucleotide excision repair (NER) pathway more closely as it repairs damage from the most common exogenous DNA-damaging agent, UVR (DiGiovanna & Kraemer, 2012).

The most common source of UVR is the sun. The skin, lips, ocular tissues, and tip of the tongue are all tissues normally exposed to UVR from the sun. UVR causes two basic types of DNA damage: cyclobutene pyrimidine dimers (CPD) and 6–4 pyrimidine-pyrimidone photoproducts (6 to 4 photoproducts). These lesions distort the DNA and cause a block in the normal replication of the cell, leading to cell death if not repaired. In some cases, polymerases can bypass the lesions. However, these polymerases can cause errors to be incorporated into the DNA, leading to mutations. UVR lesions are repaired by the NER pathway (DiGiovanna & Kraemer, 2012).

The first step in the NER repair pathway is identification. The UVR damage is first identified by two proteins, XPC and XPE. In a series of closely choreographed steps, the damage is verified by the XPA protein, the tightly wound DNA is opened by the proteins XPB (ERCC3) and XPD (ERCC2), and the CPD or 6–4 lesion is cut out by the proteins XPF (ERCC4) and XPG (ERCC5). The "hole" left in the DNA is then filled in by a DNA polymerase. The process takes between 6 and 12 hours to complete (Ciccia & Elledge, 2010; DiGiovanna & Kraemer, 2012).

The other repair pathways—base excision repair, nonhomologous and homologous end joining, intrastrand and interstrand crosslink repair, and mismatch repair—all follow these basic steps but use a plethora of different proteins to accomplish repair of the specific DNA lesions (Aparicio et al., 2014; Hsieh & Yamane, 2008; Huang & Li, 2013).

DNA is constantly under attack from countless damaging agents from both inside and outside the cell. A vigorous response from the DNA damage-response pathways is essential for this damage to be repaired to maintain overall health. When DNA damage is not successfully repaired, mutations that may lead to cancer are the consequence. Recent research has also found that certain neurodegenerative diseases and the normal aging process are a result of unrepaired DNA damage (Rizza et al., 2021).

**Essential Facts**

- DNA damage stimulates a response mechanism to repair the lesion. The repair often occurs in the gap phases of the cell cycle.
- There are multiple types of DNA damage both intrinsic to the cell and extrinsic from the environment; if the damage is not repaired the cell may die, enter a dormant state, or eventually become malignant.
- Separate repair mechanisms have evolved to resolve different types of DNA damage; these repair mechanisms or pathways are rapidly recruited to the site of damage by multiple proteins in the nucleus. There are at least six different repair pathways active against various forms of damage.

## IMMUNITY AND CANCER — THE IMMUNE SYSTEM FIGHTS BACK (TABLE 5.6)

The theory of immune surveillance for malignancy was proposed over 100 years ago; however, it wasn't until the mid-20th and early 21st centuries that the theory was experimentally confirmed (Ribatti, 2017). When the DNA damage response has failed to repair genetically abnormal cells, the immune system is the last defense against the development of malignancies. Immunosurveillance by the immune system is an ongoing process to rid the body of malignant cells before they can progress into an organized tumor, and both the adaptive and innate immune systems work collectively to clear the body of premalignant and malignant cells. When the DNA damage response is no longer adequately functioning in abnormal cells, damaged and malignant cells can continue to propagate and eventually develop the ability to evade the immune system (Chatterjee & Walker, 2017; Stephen & Hajjar, 2020).

Immunosurveillance for cancer involves three phases. The first phase, or the elimination phase, involves multiple cell types of the innate and adaptive immune systems. Since cancer cells harbor many mutations, they often present immune-stimulating antigens or tumor-specific antigens (TSA). The immune system responds to the TSA by marshalling host defenses, including cells such as CD8+ T cells and NK (natural killer) cells, and cytokines, including interferons and interleukins, to destroy early transformed cancer cells. However, not all cancer cells may be killed (Vesely et al., 2011).

Since cells in a tumor have multiple combinations of mutations that lead to different states of antigenicity, a few cells may escape

Table 5.6

**Innate and Adaptive Immune System Cells and Their Roles in Immune Surveillance**

| | Arm of Immune System | Function in Immunity | Function in Cancer Surveillance |
|---|---|---|---|
| **Neutrophil T-cell** | Innate | Recruited to infections — first line of protection against pathogens | Tumor-associated neutrophils play two roles; can inhibit tumor progression or can be tumor enhancing. |
| **Monocytes/ Macrophages** | Innate | Monocytes migrate into tissues and differentiate into macrophages: Kupffer cells in liver, Langerhans cell in skin, microglial cells in CNS; engulf and destroy pathogens. | Tumor-associated macrophages can be both pro- and anti-tumor. The tumor microenvironment, including the presence of various cytokines, influences the behavior of both neutrophils and macrophages. |
| **Eosinophils** | Innate | Defense against parasitic and fungal infections; allergic inflammation | Function in cancer unclear; may have detrimental effects on some solid tumors by stimulating tumor inhibiting T-cells; however, elevated levels of eosinophils in breast and hematologic cancers is a poor prognostic sign. |
| **Basophils** | Innate | Active in the allergic inflammation cascade and microbial infection inflammatory response | Role in cancer is unclear; however, basophils at the site of tumors may be a poor prognostic factor. |
| **Mast cells** | Innate | Also active in the allergic inflammatory cascade; help to organize initial response to pathogens | Infiltration of tumors by mast cells can lead both good and poor prognoses. They may induce apoptosis of the tumor cells or promote tumor progression by breaking down the extracellular matrix, leading to tumor invasion of surrounding tissue. |

*(continued)*

Table 5.6

**Innate and Adaptive Immune System Cells and Their roles in Immune Surveillance (*continued*)**

| Cell Type | Arm of Immune System | Function in Immunity | Function in Cancer Surveillance |
|---|---|---|---|
| **Dendritic cells** | Innate | Gatekeepers of immune system. These cells are present in most tissues and are present in high levels in lymphoid tissue. Help maintain immune tolerance to host cells. When pathogens are present, they act to present antigens to T-cells, a critical link between the innate and adaptive immune functions. | When tumors more closely resemble normal tissues, they may escape recognition by the dendric cells. Thus, the anti-tumor response by dendritic cells is dependent on other cells in the immune system. |
| **Natural killer cells** | Innate | Powerful lymphocytes whose primary function is to eliminate cells that do not identify as "self," such as pathogens | Invade and destroy tumor cells. However, cancers can use escape mechanisms to evade identification by natural killer cells. |
| **T Lymphocytes** | Adaptive | Cellular immune response active against intracellular pathogens presented by major histocompatibility complex molecules. The cells become activated to eliminate the pathogens. There is a delicate balance between stimulatory and inhibitory signals to T lymphocytes to maintain "self" tolerance and avoid autoimmunity. | Tumor antigens stimulate the development of activated T-cells. The CD8+ population of T-cells (include cytotoxic T-cells) act to eliminate cancer cells. Depending on the tumor microenvironment, T-cells can become "exhausted" and will no longer recognize tumor antigens. |

| | | | |
|---|---|---|---|
| **B Lymphocytes** | Adaptive | Humoral immune response is mediated by B lymphocytes and are present in the blood and body fluids. | Activated B lymphocytes are recruited to the tumor microenvironment and can eliminate tumor cells through secretion of tumor-specific antibodies. |
| **Immunoglobulins** | Adaptive | Immunoglobulins are produced by activated B lymphocytes and are made up of two light and two heavy chains. These chains are rearranged in countless ways to produce an antigen-specific antibody. Each B-cell produces only one type of antibody. Thus, any new antigen in the body has the potential to activate B-cells to produce an antibody. | The development of therapeutic agents using engineered antibodies targeting antigens expressed by cancer cells |

*Notes*: The cellular components of the immune system are derived from pluripotent hematopoietic stem cells (HSC) in the bone marrow. The HSCs divide to generate the common lymphoid progenitor cells (CLP) and the common myeloid progenitor cells (CMP). The CMP cells develop into cells of the innate immune system, and the CLP cells develop into the cells of the adaptive immune system.

*Source:* From Vesely, M. D., Kershaw, M. H., Schreiber, R. D., & Smyth, M. J. (2011). Natural innate and adaptive immunity to cancer. *Annual Review of Immunology*, *29*, 235–271. https://doi.org/10.1146/annurev-immunol-031210-101324.

destruction by the immune system. The equilibrium phase of the immune response results when the immune system attempts to render the tumor dormant, so it is not able to grow and/or metastasize (Vesely et al., 2011). Cancer treatments can cause tumor dormancy, whereby not all the tumor cells have been eliminated but they are no longer growing. The equilibrium phase may last months to years (Vesely et al., 2011).

Escape is the final phase and represents a failure of immune surveillance. In this phase the malignantly transformed cells have acquired sufficient mutations to completely evade the immune system. The mutilations often upregulate driver genes, such as *EGFR* (epidermal growth factor) and *MAP3K1* (mitogen-activated protein kinase 1). Tumor-suppressor genes, including *PTEN* (phosphatase and tensin homolog) or *TP53*, also may be mutated and no longer function properly. The tumor will become clinically evident if this is a new neoplasm, or a preexisting tumor will demonstrate regrowth and metastases may become detectable (Ribatti, 2017; Vesely et al., 2011).

Extensive research in mice and human cancer cell lines has demonstrated the collaborative role the innate and adaptive immune systems play in the prevention — and surprisingly — the promotion of cancer. The term "immunoediting" refers to the concept that the immune system can eliminate certain malignant cells in a tumor, while enhancing the development of other malignant cells. The surviving cells in a tumor continue to grow, develop more mutations, and become increasingly abnormal. Thus the body is protected from malignancy by the immune system, but at the same time the process of carcinogenesis can be driven by the actions of the immune system (Vesely et al., 2011).

In the process of immune surveillance and elimination, the innate and adaptive immune systems react rapidly in recognizing and eliminating abnormal cells; however, there is a dark side to this response. Cytokines and chemokines are released and damage healthy cells in the surrounding area of the tumor, setting up an inflammatory tumor microenvironment. This can become a vicious cycle resulting in chronic inflammation and increased DNA damage, further resulting in gene mutations. The inflamed tumor microenvironment can lead to additional malignant transformation of other cells and tumor progression. This state of chronic inflammation surrounding a tumor has been termed "*a wound that does not heal*" (Stephen & Hajjar, 2020). Recent research has found that the immune system can "sculpt" tumors to be more lethal by eliminating tumor cells that express certain antigens and not eliminating other tumor cells that are able to evade immune-mediated killing, leading to the growth of a more aggressive tumor (Malmberg et al., 2017; Ribatti, 2017).

## IMMUNE DYSFUNCTION AND CANCER

When the immune system is not functioning properly, either due to a congenital abnormality, immune-suppressing drugs, or infection, the risks for developing a malignancy increase. For example, solid organ transplant recipients are immune suppressed to prevent organ rejection and are at a significantly increased risk for skin cancer, especially squamous cell carcinoma. In most incidences, these types of skin tumors can be surgically removed. However, skin tumors such as melanoma and Merkel cell cancers may metastasize and lead to early mortality in transplant patients (Garrett et al., 2016).

Diseases, either genetic or acquired, can result in an abnormally functioning immune system, leading to an increased risk for malignancy. Inborn errors of immune dysfunction (primary immune deficiency disorders) are associated with immunodeficiency, autoimmune disease, and hyperinflammation. They result in infections by opportunistic organisms, including candida, mycobacteria, and an inability to control infections with EBV (Epstein Barr virus) and other commonly encountered viruses. Inborn errors of immune dysfunction also cause autoimmune diseases, including enteropathy, rheumatoid-type arthritis, thyroid dysfunction, and hematologic abnormalities, including lymphopenias, thrombocytopenia, and autoimmune anemias (Delmonte et al., 2019). Since the innate and/or adaptive arms of the immune system are dysfunctional in these diseases, this poses a significant problem for cancer surveillance and leads to an increased risk for development of malignancies. Immunodeficiency disorders, including combined variable immunodeficiency, idiopathic CD4 lymphopenia, and others, are associated with an increased risk of developing cancer (Shavit et al., 2021). AIDS (acquired immune deficiency syndrome) patients are also at an increased risk for malignancies. Virally induced Kaposi sarcoma (caused by human herpesvirus 8 [HHV-8] and non-Hodgkin lymphoma, such as Burkitt lymphoma [caused by EBV]) has been tightly associated with the diagnosis of AIDS. Women with AIDS are at significantly increased risk for invasive HPV-associated cervical cancer. Often AIDS patients present with more aggressive and advanced neoplasms (Rihana et al., 2018).

In summary, the immune system usually rids the body of tumor cells. Immunoediting is the process by which the immune system surveils, eliminates, or renders malignant cells dormant. If the immune system cannot contain the malignant cells, then tumor cells escape and progression occurs (Stephen & Hajjar, 2020; Vesely et al., 2011) Dysfunction of the immune system by genetic diseases or acquired infections can result in abnormal tumor surveillance and a higher risk for the development of malignancy. Continued understanding of the immune system's role in tumor surveillance and destruction has led to the development of cancer treatment with immunotherapy and the recent development of CAR-T cells. This will be discussed later in the chapter.

**Essential Facts**

- The immune system is the final stage in cancer prevention when the DNA damage response fails to repair DNA lesions.
- Immune surveillance is an ongoing process whereby multiple cells in both the innate and adaptive arms identify and eliminate abnormal cells. However, cancer cells can evade detection by the immune system.
- Tumor cells can impede the actions of the immune system by immunologically hiding from the immune system or by inhibiting the actions of immune cells.
- Inherited or acquired conditions limiting the function of the immune system can lead to an increased incidence of malignancy.

## GENE ENVIRONMENT INTERACTION — CARCINOGENS AND HOW THEY LEAD TO CANCER

A carcinogen is any substance that promotes the development of cancer. Scrotal cancer was the first carcinogen-related cancer to be fully described. Young boys were used as chimney sweeps in England and would accumulate coal tar and other substances in the rugae (skin) of the scrotum as they cleaned chimneys. In 1775, a London surgeon named Percival Pott reported the relationship between a relatively rare type of cancer (scrotal cancer) and a relatively rare job (chimney sweep). Although child labor was not unusual in England during the 1700s, the only young boys who developed scrotal cancer were chimney sweeps. Thus, Pott was able to connect exposure to burned coal tar chimney waste with the development of scrotal cancer in these young boys. This is an early example of cancer epidemiology. By the early 1930s, research identified multiple carcinogenic substances in the coal tar of chimney waste: benzo[a]pyrene in coal tar was found to be an especially potent carcinogen (Lipsick, 2021).

In 1908, a French physician irradiated rats after seeing reports of physicians developing cancers on their hands after performing multiple x-rays on patients. He performed these animal experiments to test whether x-rays could cause cancer. Several of the rats did indeed develop invasive tumors at the sites of irradiation. Despite these findings, x-rays were still used over the years for many doubtful non-medical reasons, including assessing how shoes fit. Additional evidence for the carcinogenic properties of x-rays came after the atomic bombing of Hiroshima and Nagasaki. Survivors of the bombing were found to develop cancer at a high rate. In 1951, Joseph Muller, an American geneticist, proposed that the cancers arose due to multiple mutations in single somatic cells caused by radiation exposure to the atomic bombs (Lipsick, 2021).

Carcinogens are, by definition, substances originating outside of the body that are capable of causing cancer. Carcinogens cause DNA damage, leading to mutations in genes important for multiple cellular activities, including cell division, DNA repair, immune regulation, and metabolism. As discussed previously, IR causes double- and single-strand DNA breaks, a particularly carcinogenic form of damage. However, IR can also cause single base-pair changes, which also lead to gene mutations (Aparicio et al., 2014). UVR from sunlight is a carcinogen that leads to DNA damage by causing bulky DNA-distorting lesions. These same types of bulky DNA-distorting lesions are also caused by some chemotherapy agents and carcinogens in cigarette smoke. Unrepaired, the lesions can result in gene mutations and cancer (Chatterjee & Walker, 2017; DiGiovanna & Kraemer, 2012).

Assessing whether a substance is carcinogenic relies on several methodologies. Laboratory analyses using bacteria, yeast, laboratory animals, and cell lines are the initial methods utilized to assess whether a substance is carcinogenic (Zhang et al., 2009). Second, epidemiology studies look at rates of cancer in populations where an exposure occurs. Since populations may be exposed to multiple substances simultaneously it can be difficult to determine which, if any, substance is carcinogenic (Raj et al., 2014). However, if research on a substance, such as IR, is found to be conclusive, it is then listed as a known carcinogen.

There are national and multinational organizations that assess the carcinogenic capabilities of substances. The International Agency for Research on Cancer (IARC) is an agency of the World Health Organization (https://www.iarc.who.int). One of its responsibilities is to identify substances that can cause cancer. The IARC has developed a classification system for labeling substances based on their ability to cause cancer.

## IRAC Classifications

Group 1: Carcinogenic to humans
Group 2A: Probably carcinogenic to humans
Group 2B: Possibly carcinogenic to humans
Group 3: Not classifiable as to its carcinogenicity in humans

The National Toxicology Program (NTP) is mandated by the U.S. Congress; it includes departments of the National Institutes of Health, the Centers for Disease Control and Prevention, and the Food and Drug Administration. The NTP publishes a yearly report reviewing the work of these various groups in assessing the safety and impact of multiple environmental exposures. The exposures they assess are diverse and include pesticide exposures and types of artificial light exposures. One of the responsibilities of this program is to publish a list of substances the NTP has identified as being carcinogenic. The NTP has a simple classification system: (1) Substances known to be human carcinogens and (2) Substances reasonably anticipated to be human carcinogens. The "14th Report on Carcinogens," published in 2016, has a comprehensive list of 248 substances considered to be carcinogenic by the NTP. However, the NTP continues to evaluate substances for their carcinogenic risk, and other substances eventually may be added to this list. The NTP website is https://ntp.niehs.nih.gov.

## Essential Facts

Common Environmental Carcinogens: This is a very small list of environmental carcinogens that may be encountered on a daily basis. A more complete list of commonly encountered and workplace carcinogens can be found at the IARC website: https://monographs.iarc.who.int/cards_page/publications-monographs

1. UVR broad spectrum from sunlight, sunlamps, and tanning beds
2. Infectious agents
   a. Chronic infection with hepatitis B and C – liver cancer
   b. Helicobacter pylori – stomach cancer
   c. Human papillomavirus – cancers of the cervix, vulva, penis, throat, rectum, anus
   d. Human T-cell lymphotropic virus type 1 (HTLV-1) – hematologic malignancies
   e. Human Immunodeficiency Virus (HIV) – cancers of cervix, anus, lung, breast, head, and neck (Chiu et al., 2017)
   f. EBV – hematologic malignancies
   g. Kaposi sarcoma–associated herpes virus – Kaposi sarcoma
   h. Merkel cell polyomavirus – Merkel cell skin cancer
3. Tobacco – including secondhand tobacco smoke. There are at least 70 known carcinogens in tobacco and cigarette smoke (www.compoundchem.com/2014/05/01/the-chemicals-in-cigarette-smoke-their-effects)

*(continued)*

*(continued)*

4. Alcohol intake is associated with cancers of the mouth, throat, larynx, esophagus, breast, liver, and colon and rectum (Guidolin et al., 2021; www.cancer.gov/about-cancer/causes-prevention/risk/alcohol/alcohol-fact-sheet)
5. Ionizing radiation:
   X-ray and gamma radiation
   Radon gas – a naturally occurring radioactive gas associated with lung cancer in nonsmokers
   Radium
6. Asbestos – Mesothelioma, a relatively rare cancer, is almost exclusively caused by asbestos exposure.

In conclusion, carcinogens are any exogenous substance capable of damaging DNA, leading to the development of cancer. Carcinogens can be encountered in the general environment and in the workplace. It often requires multiple exposures over several years for cancer to develop after a carcinogen exposure. As an example, nonmelanoma skin cancer, caused by UV radiation, is unusual in individuals under age 60 years, although people are exposed to the sun from birth. Therefore, when an individual develops skin cancer, it has taken many exposures over multiple decades for the carcinogen (UV) to cause cancer. The inherited makeup of individuals also can determine the risk for cancer after a carcinogen exposure. Individuals who have inherited more darkly pigmented skin are less likely to develop nonmelanoma skin cancer than individuals who have inherited a lighter skin pigmentation (DiGiovanna & Kraemer, 2012).

Multiple organizations and databases have been developed to track carcinogens and carcinogen exposures. As new information from clinical and epidemiological studies becomes available, the number and type of carcinogens will be clarified, enabling safer homes, medications, and workplaces.

## Essential Facts

There are multiple factors determining whether an individual develops cancer following carcinogen exposure. Elements contributing to risk for cancer development include the following:

- Amount of carcinogen contact
- Duration of carcinogen exposure
- Age at carcinogen contact

*(continued)*

(continued)

- Exposure to a combination of different carcinogens
- An individual's personal genetic makeup

A comprehensive list of environmental carcinogens can be found at https://www.cancer.gov/about-cancer/causes-prevention/risk/substances

## INHERITED RISK FOR CANCER DEVELOPMENT: A CANCER IN THE FAMILY

Inherited germline mutations in cancer predisposition genes are thought to be present in 5% to 10% of people who develop cancer. Being a carrier of a germline cancer predisposition mutation places a person at an increased risk of developing cancer at a younger age and in multiple organs. However, people with an inherited germline mutation in cancer predisposition genes may never develop cancer (Riley et al., 2012). For example, inheriting a germline mutation in the *BRCA1* gene places a woman at approximately a 40% to 87% lifetime risk of developing breast cancer (Kuchenbaecker et al., 2017), whereas the lifetime risk for a woman who does not carry a *BRCA1* mutation is approximately 13% (https://seer.cancer.gov/csr/1975_2018). Women who carry a *BRCA1* mutation often develop breast cancer at younger ages (below age 50 years) and also have a higher risk for developing cancer in the contralateral breast (Brose et al., 2002) than those without the mutation.

The cancer predisposition syndromes, such as the breast/ovarian cancer syndromes, usually occur due to germline mutations in tumor-suppressor genes. The inherited germline mutation occurs in one of the pair of alleles. The other properly functioning allele is adequate to control normal cell growth. However, if a spontaneous somatic mutation occurs in the functioning allele or if that allele is deleted or silenced, the cell no longer has a working allele. Over time, as the cell accumulates additional mutations, it may become malignant.

In 1971 Alfred Knudson studied differences in the inherited and sporadic versions of retinoblastoma, a rare malignant eye tumor in children. In the inherited version of retinoblastoma, he theorized that a child had inherited a germline mutation in one of two retinoblastoma genes at conception and had a mutated gene in every cell of the body, including the retina. The retinal malignancy occurred when the function of the other retinoblastoma gene in the retina was lost. On the other hand, a sporadic retinoblastoma occurs when, just by chance, both normal retinoblastoma genes in a retinal cell are no longer functioning. This is termed the "two hit" theory of cancer development (Knudson, 1971). Many inherited germline predisposition cancers follow this pattern of development.

From a genomic nursing standpoint, the "two hit" theory follows an autosomal dominant pattern of inheritance. The initial "first hit" is inherited in the germline and passed from parent to child. The "second hit" occurs through a spontaneous loss of function in the other allele in a somatic cell. Some family members who have inherited a germline mutation may never develop cancer. This is because there has not been a loss of the second allele, or the somatic cells with both alleles no longer functioning have not accumulated enough mutations to become malignant. It is important to remember that most cancers in the general population occur due to spontaneous somatic mutations in cells and not because of inherited germline mutations.

When performing a family history, the nurse may be alerted to the possibility of an inherited germline predisposition to cancer. The following Essential Facts box describes some common characteristics for an inherited germline predisposition to cancer (www.cancer.org/cancer/cancer-causes/genetics/family-cancer-syndromes.html).

## Essential Facts

Family/personal history suggestive of inherited risk for cancer development includes the following:

1. **Unusually early age of cancer onset (e.g., premenopausal breast cancer).**
2. Multiple primary cancers in a single individual (e.g., colorectal and endometrial cancer).
3. Bilateral cancer in paired organs or multifocal disease (e.g., bilateral breast cancer or multifocal renal cancer).
4. Clustering of the same type of cancer in close relatives (e.g., mother, daughter, and sisters with breast cancer).
5. Cancers occurring in multiple generations of a family (i.e., autosomal dominant inheritance).
6. Occurrence of rare tumors (e.g., retinoblastoma, adrenocortical carcinoma, granulosa cell tumor of the ovary, ocular melanoma, or duodenal cancer, diffuse hereditary gastric cancer).
7. Occurrence of epithelial ovarian, fallopian tube, or primary peritoneal cancer.
8. Unusual presentation of cancer (e.g., male breast cancer).
9. Uncommon tumor histology (e.g., medullary thyroid carcinoma, lobular breast cancer).

*(continued)*

*(continued)*

10. Rare cancers associated with birth defects (e.g., Wilms tumor and genitourinary abnormalities).
11. Geographic or ethnic populations known to be at high risk of hereditary cancers. Genetic testing candidates may be identified based solely on ethnicity when a strong founder effect is present in a given population (e.g., Ashkenazi heritage and *BRCA1*/*BRCA2* pathogenic variants.

Not all seemingly "cancer family predisposition" occurs due to an inherited risk. Some families may live in close proximity to each other and may be exposed to common environmental carcinogens, such as atmospheric radon (Lipsick, 2021). Family members may work in similar hazardous occupations, including asbestos mining or petrochemical plants, and be exposed to carcinogens and bring carcinogen-containing material home to family members on clothing. Obtaining more detailed information on family history and obtaining medical records is important to determine whether testing for germline mutations for a cancer predisposition syndrome is indicated (Duzkale et al., 2021; Riley et al., 2012).

If a personal or family history of cancer is suspected for an inherited predisposition to cancer, genetic testing may be indicated. The benefits of testing include diagnosis of cancers at earlier, more curable stages, prophylactic risk-reduction surgery, and notification of at-risk relatives. As an example, an inherited mutation in the *CDH1* gene confers a 30% to 80% risk for diffuse hereditary gastric cancer, often at an early age (Hampel et al., 2015). Suggested monitoring for *CDH1* carriers is yearly endoscopy with multiple biopsies of gastric mucosa. The definitive risk-reduction surgery is prophylactic gastrectomy.

It is advisable for individuals at risk for an inherited predisposition to cancer to have genetic counseling prior to the testing. Counseling provides the basis for an informed decision and also helps the person being tested understand the psychological implications of test results (Riley et al., 2012).

Genetic counseling helps individuals understand the actual test results themselves. Genetic testing by the use of DNA sequencing of cells obtained through blood, cheek, or saliva cells can often determine if a gene mutation is present (termed a *pathologic variant*) or absent (termed a *normal variant*). However, there can be test results that are ambiguous. A change in a gene may be considered a *variant of unknown significance* if it has not been associated with a cancer family, if the variant itself is not a severe mutation, like a missense mutation, or if additional laboratory testing has not been done to determine if the variant affects gene function. It is not always clear what the result means for cancer risk or how to monitor carriers, and it may cause anxiety in individuals who are found to have what is considered a *variant of unknown significance* (Hampel et al., 2015). Most commercial DNA testing laboratories use these or other similar terminology to report results. The laboratories may provide additional information on the condition and testing methodology.

In most incidences, DNA testing for cancer predisposition syndromes is performed using panel testing. Since there can be several genes associated with a specific cancer, panel testing of multiple genes at one time can both pinpoint the mutated gene and eliminate other genes. A family history of colorectal cancer is an example of the advisability of panel testing. At least six cancer predisposition syndromes are associated with an increased risk for colorectal cancer, including Lynch syndrome and autosomal dominant familial adenomatous polyposis (FAP). There are five genes associated with Lynch syndrome and one with FAP. A panel test can assess for deleterious changes (mutations) in all these genes. If a deleterious mutation is identified in a family member, other at-risk family members need only be tested for the identified mutation. Increasingly, laboratories performing testing for cancer predisposition genes test for a large array of genes, including those that may or may not be closely associated with the presenting cancer history (Riley et al., 2012). As an example, one laboratory uses a comprehensive approach and tests for eight types of cancers using a 36-gene panel (https://www.ambrygen.com/providers/oncology/test-menu). It is beyond the scope of this chapter to describe all the inherited cancer predisposition syndromes. A short representative list of common cancer predisposition syndromes is provided in Table 5.7. Many of the inherited cancer predisposition syndromes, such as the examples in Table 5.7, follow an autosomal dominant pattern of inheritance. However, there are other rarer cancer predisposition syndromes that have an autosomal recessive pattern of inheritance. These syndromes often include poor growth, signs of premature aging, and a pattern of neurodegeneration. Table 5.8 is a representative list of these cancer predisposition syndromes (Keijzers et al., 2017).

## Essential Facts

- An inherited predisposition to cancer is associated with approximately 5% to 10% of all cancer diagnoses.
- An early-age onset of cancer, malignancies in paired organs, and a family history of similar cancers that follows an autosomal

*(continued)*

*(continued)*

dominant pattern of inheritance are some of the features of an inherited predisposition to cancer.

- DNA testing for familial cancer syndromes is possible for multiple common cancers, including breast/ovarian cancer syndromes, GI and colon cancer syndromes, and some rarer inherited cancer syndromes.
- Panel testing, assessing for deleterious variants in multiple candidate genes, is becoming the most common way to perform DNA testing for inherited cancer syndromes.
- Results of DNA testing include *deleterious variant identified* (positive result), *no deleterious variant identified* (negative result), and *variant of unknown significance identified.* It may be difficult to determine how to monitor an individual with a variant of unknown significance.

Table 5.7

**Some Autosomal Dominant Inherited Cancer Predisposition Syndromes for More Common Cancers, the Known Genes, and Affected Tissues**

| Cancer Predisposition Syndrome | Gene(s) | Cancers |
|---|---|---|
| Lynch Syndromes 1 and 2 | *MLH1, MSH2, MSH6, PMS2* | Colon, endometrium, ovary, stomach, small bowel, biliary tract, urothelial, bladder |
| Breast Cancer/ Ovarian Cancer | *BRCA1, BRCA2, CHEK2, ATM, MLH1, MSH2, MSH6, PMS2, EPCAM, TP53* | Breast including male breast cancer, ovarian, prostate, pancreatic, melanoma (*BRCA2*) |
| Li-Fraumeni Syndrome | *TP53* | Adrenocortical carcinoma, breast cancer, central nervous system tumors, osteosarcomas, soft tissue sarcomas, multiple other cancers. Cancers in childhood and young adulthood. |
| Hereditary Diffuse Gastric Cancer | *CDH1* | Diffuse gastric cancer also called Signet Ring stomach carcinoma, women lobular breast cancer |

*Source:* https://www.ncbi.nlm.nih.gov/books/NBK1116.

Table 5.8

**Representative Autosomal Recessive Inherited Cancer Predisposition Syndromes, the Known Genes and Affected Tissues**

| Cancer Predisposition Syndrome | Gene(s) | Cancers |
|---|---|---|
| Xeroderma Pigmentosum | *XPA, ERCC2 (XPD), ERCC3 (XPB), XPC, ERCC4 (XPG), ERCC5 (XPF)*, polymerase Eta (*XPV*) | Skin cancer (all types), ocular surface cancer, central nervous system, hematologic malignancies, thyroid cancer |
| Nijmegen Breakage Syndrome | *NBS1* | Lymphoma, central nervous system malignancies, rhabdomyosarcoma |
| Fanconi Anemia Syndrome | At least 21 genes have been identified, including *BRCA2* | Hematologic malignancies, head and neck squamous cell carcinoma |
| Werner Syndrome | *WRN* | Sarcomas, melanoma, thyroid cancer, hematologic malignancies |

## THE NEW GENETIC LANDSCAPE OF CHEMOTHERAPY

The goals of cancer chemotherapy treatment are to eliminate cancer cells, reduce tumor growth, and alleviate pain (Cheung-Ong et al., 2013). The age of modern cancer chemotherapy dawned as the result of war. Soldiers in World War I and World War II exposed to sulfur mustard gases developed bone marrow failure and lymph node atrophy. It was then theorized that these effects might have been due to the killing of cells, and that there might be possible tumor-killing components present in some of these chemicals. Early animal studies of chemotherapy in the 1940s noted lymphoid tumor regression after administration of mustard gas extracts in some of the mice implanted with lymphoma tumors. Following the animal studies, human clinical trials using a stable nitrogen mustard compound reported short-lived remissions in non-Hodgkin's lymphoma and leukemia patients. Nitrogen mustard–derived drugs include cyclophosphamide, chlorambucil, uramustine, melphalan, and bendamustine (Cheung-Ong et al., 2013).

During the late 1940s and early 1950s, folic acid analogs were also in development. These chemicals blocked folic acid and inhibited the production of abnormal bone marrow cells associated with leukemia. The first antifolate drugs for chemotherapy use, aminopterin and methotrexate, were used to induce a short-lived remission in childhood leukemias (Farber & Diamond, 1948). The antifolate drugs were also found to be extremely effective in treating choriocarcinoma (Cheung-Ong et al., 2013). It was this early pioneering work done by multiple scientists that led to more widespread research into chemotherapy as a viable treatment for cancer.

Throughout the 1970s and 1980s the platinum-based drugs, such as cisplatin; antimetabolite drugs, including 5-fluorouracil, capecitabine, and fludarabine; and the anthracycline antibiotics, such as doxorubicin and daunorubicin, came into clinical use for hematologic and solid tumors. Etoposide and camptothecin, which are members of another class of drugs, the topoisomerase inhibitors, were also found to have potent antineoplastic properties (Cheung-Ong et al., 2013; Falzone et al., 2018). The concept of combination chemotherapy (the use of more than one chemotherapeutic agent at one time) was developed in the 1960s and 1970s; it widened the range of interaction between the drugs, simultaneously killing cells with different genetic abnormalities in the tumors. The combination treatments led to better overall responses. For example, MOPP (mechlorethamine, oncovin, procarbazine, and prednisone) achieved complete remission of over 5 years in 60% of patients with Hodgkin lymphoma (Falzone et al., 2018).

Despite the classes of chemotherapy drugs' having very different chemical compositions, they all have a common basis of activity: chemotherapy drugs severely damage DNA, resulting in the death of cancer cells. The platinum-based drugs cause intrastrand crosslinking of a DNA strand, leading to disruption of cell function and apoptosis in a dividing cell. Alkylating drugs, such as carmustine, dacarbazine, and temozolomide, cause interstrand crosslinks between the opposite strands of DNA, resulting in apoptosis of dividing cells. Other chemotherapy drugs, such as methotrexate, block the normal synthesis of nucleotides, causing DNA replication to fail (Cheung-Ong et al., 2013).

There are limitations to these chemotherapeutic drugs. First, some cells in the tumor may be resistant to the effects of the drug. This resistance may lead to a partial response to treatment with later growth of the resistant cells, resulting in recurrence of the tumor. Second, these drugs are not selective in their activity and not only damage the DNA of cancer cells, but also damage the DNA of normal healthy tissue, resulting in toxicities. For example, the anthracycline drugs damage the DNA of cardiomyocytes and can be very cardiotoxic; the platinum-based drugs can cause kidney damage and neurotoxicity through DNA damage to these organs (Cheung-Ong et al., 2013).

## GENOMIC AGENTS TO THE RESCUE

The newer targeted therapies were developed as a result of basic research in the areas of immunology, cell and molecular biology, and sequencing of the human and cancer genomes. Owing to the improved understanding of the basic genetic and molecular mechanisms behind carcinogenesis, the targeted chemotherapies are directed toward specific genetic molecular changes in cancer cells while mostly sparing normal cells. Many of these molecular targets were identified by genetic sequencing of tumors.

The Cancer Genome Atlas (TCGA) is a federally funded collaborative effort between the National Cancer Institute and the Human Genome Research Institute. The project was begun in 2006 with the goal of sequencing and cataloging mutations, proteins, and other DNA abnormalities in cells off 33 different cancer types. Information about DNA abnormalities, such as tumor mutations, interacting cellular pathways, and changes in proteins of cancer cells, are placed in the large TCGA database. This database is publicly available to cancer researchers throughout the world and has generated over 2.5 petabytes of information on multiple types of cancer data. Drug development, including molecularly targeted chemotherapy drugs, has been augmented through information contained in the TCGA database. This program has also resulted in the ability to diagnose cancer at an earlier stage and treat the condition in a more targeted approach. See https://ww.cancer.gov/about-nci/organization/ccg/research/structural-genomics/tcga.

Targeted therapeutic drugs are recombinant proteins, mostly monoclonal antibodies (immune system proteins created in a laboratory), directed toward specific cellular changes and proteins involved in cancer development and progression. The monoclonal antibodies are made through genetic engineering processes combining human and at times mouse immunoglobulins directed at specific DNA targets on cancer cells (Falzone et al., 2018). The first approved monoclonal antibody in clinical practice was rituximab. The drug targets the CD20 protein on the cell surface of both cancer and normal cells. It was found to be beneficial in the treatment of non-Hodgkin's lymphoma and was well tolerated even at higher doses. Moreover, when it was combined with a standard chemotherapy, CHOP (cyclophosphamide, hydroxydaunorubicin, vincristine, and prednisone), there was a significant improvement in outcomes for non-Hodgkin's lymphoma patients (Falzone et al., 2018). A year later, trastuzumab (Herceptin), a monoclonal antibody directed toward the (*HER2*)/neu receptor, was FDA approved. The antibody blocks the *HER2* receptor, resulting in eventual cell death. Herceptin is used to treat HER+ breast and gastric cancers (Tariman, 2017). Additional monoclonal antibody drugs were developed as new "drug able" molecular targets were identified. Since the approval of trastuzumab and rituximab many other monoclonal antibody drugs have been developed.

Enzyme inhibitory drugs are monoclonal antibodies that have been developed through basic research into pathways important to the abnormal growth and proliferation of cancer cells. The concept of enzyme inhibitory drugs is not new. For example, the antibiotics penicillin and vancomycin are enzyme inhibitory drugs that interfere with the growth of bacterial cell walls, resulting in killing of the bacteria (Katz & Caufield, 2003). Small molecule drugs directed against cancer more easily enter cancer cells and inhibit abnormal cell growth. Examples of small molecule inhibitors include Ruxolitimib, Sorafenib, and Everolimus. Ruxolitimib is a janus kinase inhibitor used to treat hematologic malignancies such as myelofibrosis. Sorafenib is a tyrosine kinase inhibitor used to treat multiple types of solid tumors, including kidney and liver cancer. Recently, it was the first drug approved to treat plexiform neurofibromas, a particularly devastating consequence of NFI (neurofibromatosis type 1) (Kim et al., 2013). Everolimus is an mTOR pathway inhibitor that is used to treat breast, kidney, and pancreatic cancers. It is a versatile drug and can also be used to prevent rejection of organ transplants and treat seizures related to tuberous sclerosis. These small molecule drugs all inhibit different pathways in cells but result in the disruption of vital growth pathways, leading to treatment of cancer and other conditions (Falzone et al., 2018).

In 2017 the FDA issued regulatory guidelines for the development of new cancer drugs, including the monoclonal antibody–derived drugs. The guidelines included regulations for basic drug development in laboratories, clinical experimentation (animal studies and clinical trials in patients), the approval process, and commercialization and marketing for chemotherapy and monoclonal antibody drugs. The guidelines cover all stages of drug development. The guidelines stated that the non-clinical studies should elucidate the prime activity of the drug, for example what pathway is being targeted. There should be testing in animal models to initially assess effectiveness and toxicities. Specific clinical trials need to be conducted in patients who have the tumor of interest. These clinical trials for patients should assess the pharmacokinetics, clearance, activity, and the patients' responses to the drug (Falzone et al., 2018).

## IMMUNE PATHWAYS FOR DRUG DEVELOPMENT

Recently, the power of the immune system to identify and kill malignant cells has been harnessed in the development of new immunotherapy agents. As was discussed previously, the cells of the adaptive immune system, such as the CD4+ T-cell and CD8+ T- and B-cells, identify and destroy malignant cells. They are immensely powerful against both pathogens and malignant cells. When an infectious organism or malignancy develops, antigens on the surface of the infecting agent or tumor interact with the major histocompatibility complex and antigen-presenting cells (APC). Through a complex process, the APC activates the T-cells that then initiate killing of the infectious organism or tumor cells. However, it is important to have negative (protective) regulation to prevent T-cells from attacking normal tissue. One of the pathways critical for protecting healthy tissue from the adaptive immune system is the cytotoxic T lymphocyte antigen 4 (CTLA4) inhibitory pathway. CTLA4 is a receptor on the surface of T-cells. When it is activated, the CTLA4 pathway inhibits T-cells and stops their proliferation, interrupting the immune response (Alegre et al., 2001). The ability to stop T-cell activation against normal tissue is termed a checkpoint. Cancer cells take advantage of this checkpoint to evade T-cells. The first checkpoint inhibitory drug, ipilimumab (a human IgG monoclonal antibody), binds to and blocks the CTLA4 receptors on the T-cells; with the CTLA4 receptors blocked, the T-cells can recognize, proliferate, and attack the tumor cells (Falzone et al., 2018).

The PD1/PDL-1 immune pathway is also being exploited for use in cancer treatment. As with the CTLA4 pathway, the PD1/PD-L1 pathway protects healthy tissue from the innate immune system — termed peripheral T-cell tolerance. Normally, when the PD-L1 binds the PD-1 found on T-cells it prevents the T-cells from killing the healthy cells. However, the PD-L1 receptor may be overexpressed by cancer cells so they can "hide" from the T-cells, allowing the cancer to progress (Sharpe & Pauken, 2018). Recently, new drugs targeting the PD-1/PD-L1 pathway have been developed and include pembrolizumab and nivolumab, which block PD-1, and atezolizumab, avelumab, and durvalumab, which block PD-L1. Research has found that blocking of the PD-1/PD-L1 signaling pathway significantly enhances antitumor immunity, produces durable clinical responses, and prolongs survival in some cancer patients. The PD-1/PD-L1 drugs are most effective against tumor cells with many mutations, as those tumors tend to produce more antigenic proteins, which alert the immune system (Akinleye & Rasool, 2019).

Both the CTLA4 and PD-1/PDL-1 blockade drugs are well tolerated; however, they can have serious immune-related toxicities. The toxicities can be mild, such as skin rashes treated with topical steroid creams, to life-threatening events, such as autoimmune encephalitis, pneumonitis, and nephritis.. These toxicities are directly related to the drugs' action of inhibiting the pathways that normally keep the immune system in check, protecting normal tissues. Some of these immune toxicities can be dealt with by temporary cessation of the drug, but at times the more severe toxicities require total termination of the drug and treatment with potent corticosteroids. The more serious toxicities can be seen in combination use of both CTLA4 and PD-1/PDL-1 drugs (Sharpe & Pauken, 2018).

Car-T cell therapy is a new particularly powerful treatment for hematologic cancers. Car (chimeric antigen receptor) T-cells are T-cells that have been genetically modified in a laboratory to target specific surface antigens of tumor cells. The modified T-cells are infused back into the patient, and the modified T-cells target and kill tumor cells containing the specific antigen (Li et al., 2020). The most serious complication of Car-T cell therapy is cytokine release syndrome (CRS). Signs of CRS include high fever, lethargy, myalgia, tachycardia, hypotension, capillary leakage, cardiac and renal damage, liver failure, and DIC (disseminated intravascular coagulation). The cause of CRS is the excessive release of cytokines, including $INF_{y}$, IL6, IL1, and IL2RA. These cytokines are released by the Car-T cells in response to interaction with tumor antigens. The CRS normally occurs approximately 1 to 2 weeks after therapy. CRS is treated with either cetuximab or tocilizumab and glucocorticoids to calm the runaway immune response. CRS can be relatively mild or severe necessitating ICU admission and can be lethal (Li et al., 2020). CRS is an expected event after Car-T cell therapy and may indicate effectiveness of the treatment. The severity of CRS currently limits the usefulness of Car-T cells in solid tumors. Since Car-T cells are a powerful personalized immunotherapy, there is ongoing research into the management of CRS to further the use of Car-T cells in cancer treatment (Brandt et al., 2020).

New targeted and immunotherapy drugs are continually in development. For a comprehensive list of targeted and immunotherapy chemotherapy agents that are in common clinical use, Nursing Clinic of North America (Tariman, 2017).

## Essential Facts

- The development of cancer chemotherapy began in the 1940s and 1950s and includes drugs still commonly in use.
- Although chemotherapy drugs use different mechanisms, the primary mode of action is to severely damage cancer cell DNA, resulting in cell death and tumor reduction.
- Research in the disciplines of immunology, cell and molecular biology, and genetics has led to the development of new highly effective targeted and immunotherapy agents and Car-T cell therapy, which harness the power of the immune system to kill tumor cells.

## CONCLUSION

Cancer is an old disease; signs of cancer have been detected in dinosaurs. Egyptian physicians were the first to specifically describe the condition, and evidence of the disease has been found in mummies. Throughout the ensuing millennia, cancer was a uniformly fatal condition. It wasn't until the development of improved sterile surgical procedures and effective anesthesia in the early 20th century that the safe surgical removal of solid tumors was possible. However, metastatic disease and cancers of the blood-forming organs were still lethal. The modern age of cancer treatment dawned with the use of radiation and chemotherapy in the mid-20th century. People with cancer received improved therapies and lived longer with their disease. However, it was still difficult to exact a cure.

The age of molecular medicine dawned because of research from a combination of many basic sciences, including chemistry, cell biology, genetics, pharmacology, and immunology. The understanding that cancers were caused by gene mutations and that certain mutations were important for cancer growth allowed the development of drugs targeting these specific cellular changes and gene mutations. In the past several years, immunology research of cancer has opened the door to new drugs, allowing the immune system to actively target and destroy cancer cells. The development of new genetic technologies continues to aid research that detects ways to target gene mutations and molecular pathways for improved treatment of cancer patients.

## END-OF-CHAPTER QUESTIONS

1. In which phase of the cell cycle does the cell copy or synthesize DNA?
2. Name one type of chromosome abnormality commonly seen in cancer cells.
3. In which step of carcinogenesis is a cell considered to be a precancer?
4. Which type of gene acts as a "brake" on cell division and tumor development?
5. Which type of DNA damage is devastating for a cell and is utilized in radiation therapy for cancer?
6. What percentage of cancer deaths result from metastasis?
7. Which DNA repair pathway is responsible for repairing sunlight-induced DNA damage?
8. Name the two arms of the immune system.
9. Which type of immune cell is in the first line of protection from pathogens and tumor cells?

10. What percentage of people who develop a malignancy cancer have an inherited predisposition to cancer?
11. Name one inherited cancer predisposition syndrome.
12. Which chemical weapons used in World Wars I and II led to the development of the first chemotherapy agents?
13. What was the first monoclonal antibody therapeutic agent?
14. Which immune pathway is targeted by pembrolizumab?

## VIGNETTES

### A Tale of Two Melanomas:

In 2018, almost 84,000 cases of melanoma were diagnosed and over eight thousand people died from melanoma. U.S. Cancer Statistics Working Group. U.S. Cancer Statistics Data Visualizations Tool, based on 2020 submission data (1999–2018): U.S. Department of Health and Human Services, Centers for Disease Control and Prevention and National Cancer Institute; www.cdc.gov/cancer/dataviz, released in June 2021.

The development of melanoma is associated with exposures to common environmental carcinogens, including UV from the sun and cigarette smoking. Having a family history of melanoma, especially in a first-degree relative, doubles the risk for developing the condition (Zocchi et al., 2021).

#### *Patient Vignette 1*

MK is a 42-year-old male who lives in Madison, Wisconsin. He was a 19-year, two pack a day smoker but quit approximately 3 years ago. MK works as an arc welder and is very scrupulous in using shielding. However, he has had some facial burns. He enjoys fishing of all sorts and has traveled to the Gulf Coast of Florida on fishing trips; he is an intermittent user of sunscreens. MK has many moles on his trunk, arms, and legs. His wife noticed a "dark mole" on his posterior right shoulder was enlarging and urged her husband to see a dermatologist. On exam, the mole was considered suspicious: asymmetrically shaped, the borders were irregular, parts of the mole were darker than others, and the mole measured 5 mm in diameter and per the patient's history the mole was changing over several months' time. A biopsy of the lesion reported a stage 2 malignant melanoma; the tumor had penetrated the epidermis and had extended to the dermis. MK underwent a sentinel node biopsy, which was negative. A sentinel node biopsy is a procedure to determine if cancer cells have metastasized to the regional lymph nodes, draining the area of the tumor.

MK had an additional wide excision surgery of the lesional area, and all surgical margins were clear. He was instructed on strict UV protection and underwent close dermatology monitoring for melanoma reoccurrence over the next 5 years.

His family history was negative for melanoma; however, MK's maternal uncle had died at age 74 from pancreatic cancer. His mother was a heavy smoker who died from lung cancer at age 41. Two years after his initial diagnosis, MK was diagnosed with two new primary melanomas, one on his right calf, the other on his left anterior forearm. Both melanomas were in situ (superficial) and were surgically removed with clear margins on re-excision. Given MK's family history of pancreatic cancer and lung cancer and his personal history of three primary melanomas, he was recommended to undergo genetic testing for familial melanoma. Following genetic counseling MK had panel testing for mutations in seven high-penetrant familial melanoma genes. MK was found to have a deleterious mutation in the tumor-suppressor gene *CDKN2A*. Most hereditary melanoma families have mutations in *CDKN2A*. It was recommended that MK have screening for both pancreatic and lung cancer in addition to melanoma skin cancer screening. Being a carrier for mutations in *CDKN2A* is associated with an increased risk for pancreatic and lung cancer (Zocchi et al., 2021).

### *Patient Vignette 2*

SS is a 33-year-old female. She works as a computer software developer in Seattle, Washington. She is originally from Ogden, Utah, and is an avid skier and snowboarder. As a teenager she would use tanning booths on a semi-regular basis — at least six times a year. She is pregnant with her second child, and at a routine prenatal exam the nurse-midwife noted an unusual looking mole on SS's right lateral neck. The patient stated the mole had "always been there." However, the nurse-midwife referred SS to a dermatologist for further evaluation. The mole was 4 mm in diameter and very irregularly shaped; in addition, it had several gradations of color from pale to dark brown. A biopsy was performed, and the pathology identified a melanoma-in-situ. A re-excision of the lesion was performed, and all margins were clear. SS underwent close dermatologic monitoring during the rest of her pregnancy and will be followed closely by dermatology for the next 5 years.

The patient's family history was positive for melanoma in her father. He developed an invasive melanoma on his left lateral flank at 61. The melanoma was stage IV (the tumor had invaded the deep tissues to >4 mm) and the sentinel node biopsy identified five positive lymph nodes. A subsequent metastatic evaluation identified three sites of tumor in the left lung. The tumor had a high mutational burden (large number of somatic mutations in a tumor). He is currently undergoing treatment with an immune checkpoint inhibitor (pembrolizumab). There are no other cases of cancer in the family. However, SS was very concerned about cancer risk to her three siblings and her children and requested to undergo genetic testing for familial melanoma. She had testing for seven high-risk familial melanoma genes, and no deleterious mutations were found. However, the full genetic basis of most melanoma development susceptibility remains under investigation, and there may be other yet unidentified genes. In addition, both inherited and environmental factors contribute to melanoma development. SS will continue to undergo recommended monitoring for melanoma due to her personal history. However, no additional recommendations will currently be made for her children or siblings outside of UV protection and routine skin exams (Zocchi et al., 2021).

## REFERENCES

Akinleye, A., & Rasool, Z. (2019). Immune checkpoint inhibitors of PD-L1 as cancer therapeutics. *Journal of Hematology & Oncology, 12*(1), 92. https://doi.org/10.1186/s13045-019-0779-5

Alegre, M. L., Frauwirth, K. A., & Thompson, C. B. (2001). T-cell regulation by CD28 and CTLA-4. *Nature Reviews Immunology, 1*(3), 220–228. https://doi.org/10.1038/35105024

Aparicio, T., Baer, R., & Gautier, J. (2014). DNA double-strand break repair pathway choice and cancer. *DNA Repair, 19*, 169–175. https://doi.org/10.1016/j.dnarep.2014.03.014

Brandt, L. J. B., Barnkob, M. B., Michaels, Y. S., Heiselberg, J., & Barington, T. (2020). Emerging approaches for regulation and control of CAR T cells: A mini review. *Frontiers in Immunology, 11*, 326. https://doi.org/10.3389/fimmu.2020.00326

Branzei, D., & Foiani, M. (2008). Regulation of DNA repair throughout the cell cycle. *Nature Reviews Molecular Cell Biology, 9*(4), 297–308. https://doi.org/10.1038/nrm2351

Brose, M. S., Rebbeck, T. R., Calzone, K. A., Stopfer, J. E., Nathanson, K. L., & Weber, B. L. (2002). Cancer risk estimates for BRCA1 mutation carriers identified in a risk evaluation program. *Journal of the National Cancer Institute, 94*(18), 1365–1372. https://doi.org/10.1093/jnci/94.18.1365

Chatterjee, N., & Walker, G. C. (2017). Mechanisms of DNA damage, repair, and mutagenesis. *Environmental and Molecular Mutagenesis, 58*(5), 235–263. https://doi.org/10.1002/em.22087

Cheung-Ong, K., Giaever, G., & Nislow, C. (2013). DNA-damaging agents in cancer chemotherapy: Serendipity and chemical biology. *Chemistry & Biology, 20*(5), 648–659. https://doi.org/10.1016/j.chembiol.2013.04.007

Chiu, C. G., Smith, D., Salters, K. A., Zhang, W., Kanters, S., Milan, D., & Wiseman, S. M. (2017). Overview of cancer incidence and mortality among people living with HIV/AIDS in British Columbia, Canada: Implications for HAART use and NADM development. *BMC Cancer, 17*(1), 270. https://doi.org/10.1186/s12885-017-3229-1

Ciccia, A., & Elledge, S. J. (2010). The DNA damage response: Making it safe to play with knives. *Molecular Cell, 40*(2), 179–204. https://doi.org/10.1016/j.molcel.2010.09.019

Delmonte, O. M., Castagnoli, R., Calzoni, E., & Notarangelo, L. D. (2019). Inborn errors of immunity with immune dysregulation: From bench to bedside. *Frontiers in Pediatrics, 7*, 353. https://doi.org/10.3389/fped.2019.00353

DiGiovanna, J. J., & Kraemer, K. H. (2012). Shining a light on xeroderma pigmentosum. *Journal of Investigative Dermatology, 132*(3 Pt 2), 785–796. https://doi.org/10.1038/jid.2011.426

Duzkale, N., Oz, O., Turkmenoglu, T. T., Cetinkaya, K., Eren, T., & Yalcin, S. (2021). Investigation of hereditary cancer predisposition genes of patients with colorectal cancer: Single-centre experience. *Journal of College of Physicians and Surgeons Pakistan, 30*(7), 811–816. https://doi.org/10.29271/jcpsp.2021.07.811

Falzone, L., Salomone, S., & Libra, M. (2018). Evolution of cancer pharmacological treatments at the turn of the third millennium. *Frontiers in Pharmacology, 9*, 1300. https://doi.org/10.3389/fphar.2018.01300

Farber, S., & Diamond, L. K. (1948). Temporary remissions in acute leukemia in children produced by folic acid antagonist, 4-aminopteroyl-glutamic acid. *New England Journal of Medicine, 238*(23), 787–793. https://doi.org/10.1056/NEJM194806032382301

Fearon, E. R., & Vogelstein, B. (1990). A genetic model for colorectal tumorigenesis. *Cell, 61*(5), 759–767. https://doi.org/10.1016/0092-8674(90)90186-i

Garrett, G. L., Lowenstein, S. E., Singer, J. P., He, S. Y., & Arron, S. T. (2016). Trends of skin cancer mortality after transplantation in the United States: 1987 to 2013. *Journal of the American Academy of Dermatology, 75*(1), 106–112. https://doi.org/10.1016/j.jaad.2016.02.1155

Guidolin, V., Carlson, E. S., Carra, A., Villalta, P. W., Maertens, L. A., Hecht, S. S., & Balbo, S. (2021). Identification of new markers of alcohol-derived DNA damage in humans. *Biomolecules, 11*(3). https://doi.org/10.3390/biom11030366

Hampel, H., Bennett, R. L., Buchanan, A., Pearlman, R., Wiesner, G. L., Guideline Development Group, American College of Medical Genetics and Genomics Professional Practice and Guidelines Committee, & National Society of Genetic Counselors Practice Guidelines Committee. (2015). A practice guideline from the American College of Medical Genetics and Genomics and the National Society of Genetic Counselors: Referral indications for cancer predisposition assessment. *Genetics in Medicine, 17*(1), 70–87. https://doi.org/10.1038/gim.2014.147

Harbers, L., Agostini, F., Nicos, M., Poddighe, D., Bienko, M., & Crosetto, N. (2021). Somatic copy number alterations in human cancers: An analysis of publicly available data from the cancer genome atlas. *Frontiers in Oncology, 11*, 700568. https://doi.org/10.3389/fonc.2021.700568

Hsieh, P., & Yamane, K. (2008). DNA mismatch repair: Molecular mechanism, cancer, and ageing. *Mechanisms of Ageing and Development, 129*(7–8), 391–407. https://doi.org/10.1016/j.mad.2008.02.012

Huang, Y., & Li, L. (2013). DNA crosslinking damage and cancer — A tale of friend and foe. *Translational Cancer Research, 2*(3), 144–154. https://doi.org/10.3978/j.issn.2218-676X.2013.03.01

Katz, A. H., & Caufield, C. E. (2003). Structure-based design approaches to cell wall biosynthesis inhibitors. *Current Pharmaceutical Design, 9*(11), 857–866. https://doi.org/10.2174/1381612033455305

Keijzers, G., Bakula, D., & Scheibye-Knudsen, M. (2017). Monogenic diseases of DNA repair. *New England Journal of Medicine, 377*(19), 1868–1876. https://doi.org/10.1056/NEJMra1703366

Kim, A., Dombi, E., Tepas, K., Fox, E., Martin, S., Wolters, P., … Widemann, B. C. (2013). Phase I trial and pharmacokinetic study of sorafenib in children with neurofibromatosis type I and plexiform neurofibromas. *Pediatric Blood & Cancer, 60*(3), 396–401. https://doi.org/10.1002/pbc.24281

Knudson, A. G., Jr. (1971). Mutation and cancer: Statistical study of retinoblastoma. *Proceedings of the National Academy of Sciences of the United States of America, 68*(4), 820–823. https://doi.org/10.1073/pnas.68.4.820

Kou, F., Wu, L., Ren, X., & Yang, L. (2020). Chromosome abnormalities: New insights into their clinical significance in cancer. *Molecular Therapy — Oncolytics, 17*, 562–570. https://doi.org/10.1016/j.omto.2020.05.010

Kuchenbaecker, K. B., Hopper, J. L., Barnes, D. R., Phillips, K. A., Mooij, T. M., Roos-Blom, M. J., … Olsson, H. (2017). Risks of breast, ovarian, and contralateral breast cancer for BRCA1 and BRCA2 mutation carriers. *JAMA, 317*(23), 2402–2416. https://doi.org/10.1001/jama.2017.7112

Li, W., Wu, L., Huang, C., Liu, R., Li, Z., Liu, L., & Shan, B. (2020). Challenges and strategies of clinical application of CAR-T therapy in the treatment of tumors—a narrative review. *Annals of Translational Medicine, 8*(17), 1093. https://doi.org/10.21037/atm-20-4502

Lipsick, J. (2021). A history of cancer research: Carcinogens and mutagens. *Cold Spring Harbor Perspectives in Medicine, 11*(3). https://doi.org/10.1101/cshperspect.a035857

Malmberg, K. J., Carlsten, M., Bjorklund, A., Sohlberg, E., Bryceson, Y. T., & Ljunggren, H. G. (2017). Natural killer cell-mediated immunosurveillance of human cancer. *Seminars in Immunology, 31*, 20–29. https://doi.org/10.1016/j.smim.2017.08.002

Mao, Z., Ke, Z., Gorbunova, V., & Seluanov, A. (2012). Replicatively senescent cells are arrested in G1 and G2 phases. *Aging, 4*(6), 431–435. https://doi.org/10.18632/aging.100467

Nachman, M. W., & Crowell, S. L. (2000). Estimate of the mutation rate per nucleotide in humans. *Genetics, 156*(1), 297–304. https://www.ncbi.nlm.nih.gov/pmc/articles/PMC1461236/pdf/10978293.pdf

Peitzsch, C., Tyutyunnykova, A., Pantel, K., & Dubrovska, A. (2017). Cancer stem cells: The root of tumor recurrence and metastases. *Seminars in Cancer Biology, 44*, 10–24. https://doi.org/10.1016/j.semcancer.2017.02.011

Raj, P., Hohenadel, K., Demers, P. A., Zahm, S. H., & Blair, A. (2014). Recent trends in published occupational cancer epidemiology research: Results from a comprehensive review of the literature. *American Journal of Industrial Medicine, 57*(3), 259–264. https://doi.org/10.1002/ajim.22280

Ravi, D., & Das, K. C. (2004). Redox-cycling of anthracyclines by thioredoxin system: Increased superoxide generation and DNA damage. *Cancer Chemotherapy and Pharmacology, 54*(5), 449–458. https://doi.org/10.1007/s00280-004-0833-y

Ribatti, D. (2017). The concept of immune surveillance against tumors. The first theories. *Oncotarget, 8*(4), 7175–7180. https://doi.org/10.18632/oncotarget.12739

Rihana, N., Nanjappa, S., Sullivan, C., Velez, A. P., Tienchai, N., & Greene, J. N. (2018). Malignancy trends in HIV-infected patients over the past 10 years in a single-center retrospective observational study in the United States. *Cancer Control, 25*(1), 1073274818797955. https://doi.org/10.1177/1073274818797955

Riley, B. D., Culver, J. O., Skrzynia, C., Senter, L. A., Peters, J. A., Costalas, J. W., … Trepanier, A. M. (2012). Essential elements of genetic cancer risk assessment, counseling, and testing: Updated recommendations of the National Society of Genetic Counselors. *Journal of Genetic Counseling, 21*(2), 151–161. https://doi.org/10.1007/s10897-011-9462-x

Rizza, E. R. H., DiGiovanna, J. J., Khan, S. G., Tamura, D., Jeskey, J. D., & Kraemer, K. H. (2021). Xeroderma pigmentosum: A model for human premature aging. *Journal of Investigative Dermatology, 141*(4S), 976–984. https://doi.org/10.1016/j.jid.2020.11.012

Rogalla, S., Contag, C. H. (2015). Early Cancer Detection at the Epithelial Surface. *Cancer J. 21*, 179–187.

Sharpe, A. H., & Pauken, K. E. (2018). The diverse functions of the PD1 inhibitory pathway. *Nature Reviews Immunology, 18*(3), 153–167. https://doi.org/10.1038/nri.2017.108

Shavit, R., Maoz-Segal, R., Frizinsky, S., Haj-Yahia, S., Offengenden, I., Machnas-Mayan, D., … Agmon-Levin, N. (2021). Combined immunodeficiency (CVID and CD4 lymphopenia) is associated with a high risk of malignancy among adults with primary immune deficiency. *Clinical & Experimental Immunology, 204*(2), 251–257. https://doi.org/10.1111/cei.13579

Stanbridge, E. J. (1990). Human tumor suppressor genes. *Annual Review of Genetics, 24*, 615–657. https://doi.org/10.1146/annurev.ge.24.120190.003151

Stephen, B., & Hajjar, J. (2020). Overview of basic immunology and clinical application. *Advances in Experimental Medicine and Biology, 1244*, 1–36. https://doi.org/10.1007/978-3-030-41008-7_1

Tariman, J. D. (2017). Changes in cancer treatment: Mabs, mibs, mids, nabs, and nibs. *Nursing Clinics of North America, 52*(1), 65–81. https://doi.org/10.1016/j.cnur.2016.10.004

Tessema, M., Lehmann, U., & Kreipe, H. (2004). Cell cycle and no end. *Virchows Archiv, 444*(4), 313–323. https://doi.org/10.1007/s00428-003-0971-3

Vesely, M. D., Kershaw, M. H., Schreiber, R. D., & Smyth, M. J. (2011). Natural innate and adaptive immunity to cancer. *Annual Review of Immunology, 29*, 235–271. https://doi.org/10.1146/annurev-immunol-031210-101324

Walcher, L., Kistenmacher, A. K., Suo, H., Kitte, R., Dluczek, S., Strauss, A., … Kossatz-Boehlert, U. (2020). Cancer stem cells—origins and biomarkers: Perspectives for targeted personalized therapies. *Frontiers in Immunology, 11*, 1280. https://doi.org/10.3389/fimmu.2020.01280

Wallace, S. S., Murphy, D. L., & Sweasy, J. B. (2012). Base excision repair and cancer. *Cancer Letters, 327*(1–2), 73–89. https://doi.org/10.1016/j.canlet.2011.12.038

Zhang, R., Niu, Y., Du, H., Cao, X., Shi, D., Hao, Q., & Zhou, Y. (2009). A stable and sensitive testing system for potential carcinogens based on DNA damage-induced gene expression in human HepG2 cell. *Toxicology in Vitro, 23*(1), 158–165. https://doi.org/10.1016/j.tiv.2008.10.006

Zhou, W. M., Liu, B., Shavandi, A., Li, L., Song, H., & Zhang, J. Y. (2021). Methylation landscape: Targeting writer or eraser to discover anti-cancer drug. *Frontiers in Pharmacology, 12*, 690057. https://doi.org/10.3389/fphar.2021.690057

Zocchi, L., Lontano, A., Merli, M., Dika, E., Nagore, E., Quaglino, P., … Ribero, S. (2021). Familial melanoma and susceptibility genes: A review of the most common clinical and dermoscopic phenotypic aspect, associated malignancies and practical tips for management. *Journal of Clinical Medicine, 10*(16). https://doi.org/10.3390/jcm10163760

# 6

# Genetic Assessment

Kimberly A. Subasic

*In accordance with family history and genetic testing, the physical appearance, or phenotype, of a genetic illness guides diagnosis. Some genetic illnesses have characteristic phenotypes, while others fall under the diagnostic terminology of a syndrome. Genetic illnesses that are labeled as a syndrome tend to have multiple variations in symptom presentation. This chapter will provide a brief overview of physical findings during a head-to-toe assessment that should trigger concern for a genetic association and generate further investigation by the healthcare provider.*

**In this chapter, you will learn to:**

1. Understand genomic terminology when discussing genetic illness.
2. Describe assessment findings that correlate with genetic alterations.
3. Identify red-flag genetic assessment findings.

## GENOMIC TERMINOLOGY ASSOCIATED WITH PHYSICAL ASSESSMENT

The *genotype* of a genetic disorder is its location within our DNA. Think of it as an address for where we would find this genetic misalignment. Assessment findings that are commonly associated with a particular genetic disorder are referred to the *phenotype.* This is how the disorder visually presents itself. Phenotypes help to identify and characterize specific genetic disorders. *Expressivity* is a term that describes the variation in the presentation of a specific genetic disorder. For example, there are characteristic phenotypes associated with Down syndrome, but there is a wide range of expressivity among those with this genetic alteration. The degree to which a genetic disorder is carried from generation to generation is referred to as *penetrance.* In some cases, knowledge of penetrance allows the individual and family, and the healthcare provider, to be proactive in planning for future needs.

Example: Huntington's disease has a 100% penetrance, indicating that if the individual has the genotype associated with Huntington's disease, they will eventually present with signs and symptoms associated with this disorder. Knowing the inheritance pattern (autosomal dominant) of this disorder, a genetic risk assessment should be performed for those who have other family members diagnosed with this disorder. A genetic test can confirm the presence or absence of the genotype. If the individual is genetically diagnosed with Huntington's disease, they will, with eventual certainty, present with symptoms of the illness. The phenotype of Huntington's disease consists of neuromuscular presentation of jerky movements of the arms and legs, and cognitive impairments that begin to present in middle-adulthood. Confirmation of this diagnosis will require a multifaceted, proactive approach with regard to healthcare, employment, and activities of daily living to maximize quality of life as the disease progresses.

According to Smith, Smith and del Campo (2022), *dysmorphology* is the term to describe variations that exist in the shape or structure of an expected assessment finding, whereas an *anomaly* is different than what is an expected finding. Anomalies are further described as being a major or minor anomaly based upon the functional limitations it imposes. Malformations are abnormalities that tend to occur during gestation as the cells and tissue are growing. A *syndrome* tends to suggest that the genetic disorder has multiple components to its symptom presentation. Syndromes tend to have physical assessment findings that occur across many body systems.

**Essential Facts**

Approximately 25 to 30 million Americans are considered to have a rare genetic disorder (National Institutes of Health [NIH], 2022a).

## PHYSICAL ASSESSMENT

It is critical that detailed medical family history, a *genogram*, is completed and that it extends three generations. Often, the discoveries from the genogram will guide the healthcare provider to perform a focused physical exam. Physical assessment findings that suggest genetic involvement serve as a starting point and suggest that further investigation is warranted. A list of physical assessments findings and their correlation to a genetic disorder or syndrome, located in Table 6.1, were adapted from Jones, Jones & del Campo (2022) and the National Library of Medicine, Medline Plus Genetic Conditions at https://medlineplus.gov/genetics/condition. This list, while not inclusive of all genetic disorders, provides typical assessment findings associated with genetic conditions that are more common. The association of one physical finding to a genetic disorder typically does not constitute the diagnosis of the illness. Rather, it is a comprehensive evaluation that includes a detailed family history, a thorough physical exam, and a detailed review of the person's health history, and genetic testing that yields an accurate diagnosis.

Our understanding of the human genome continues to expand. Websites such as Medline Plus Genetic Conditions (National Library of Medicine & Medline Plus, 2022) and the Genetic and Rare Diseases Information Center (National Institutes of Health, 2022b) are good sites to explore for the most up to date information on genetic findings.

Table 6.1

| Body system | Associated Genetic Disorder or Syndrome |
|---|---|
| **Neurological** | |
| Developmental delays (motor or cognitive) | Krabbe disease, Angelman syndrome, Klinefelter syndrome, Fragile X syndrome, Menkes syndrome, Smith-Lemli-Opitz syndrome, Wolf-Hirschhorn syndrome |
| Intellectual disability | Cri-du-chat Syndrome, Edwards syndrome, Patau syndrome, Hurler syndrome, Phenylketonuria, Galactosemia, Angelman syndrome, Fragile X syndrome, fetal alcohol syndrome, Williams syndrome, Prader-Willi syndrome, Coffin-Lawry syndrome, Wolf-Hirschhorn syndrome |
| Early-onset cognitive decline (adult) | Early-onset Alzheimer's disease, Huntington's disease |
| Parasthesias/Neuropathy | Gitelman syndrome, spinocerebellar ataxia |
| Seizures | Angelman syndrome |

| Body system | Associated Genetic Disorder or Syndrome |
|---|---|
| **Head and Neck** | |
| Microcephaly | Cri-du-chat syndrome, Fetal alcohol syndrome, Angelman syndrome, Smith-Lemli-Opitz syndrome, Coffin-Lowry syndrome, Rett syndrome, Wolf-Hirschhorn syndrome |
| Macrocephaly | Neurofibromatosis |
| Broad or prominent forehead | Williams syndrome, Fragile X syndrome, Coffin-Lowry syndrome, Robinow syndrome, Wolf-Hirschhorn syndrome |
| Narrow forehead | Prader-Willi syndrome |
| Premature fusion of skull, bulging forehead | Jackson-Weiss syndrome, Apert syndrome, Crouzen syndrome |
| Depressed face | Apert syndrome, Stickler syndrome |
| Long and narrow face | Fragile X syndrome |
| Small chin | Edwards syndrome |
| Large or coarse facial features | Angelman syndrome, Hurler syndrome, Smith-Lemli-Opitz syndrome, Coffin-Lowry syndrome |
| Short neck | Turner syndrome, Noonan syndrome, down Syndrome |
| Extra skin/web-like neck | Turner syndrome, Noonan syndrome |
| **Ears** | |
| Large ears | Fragile X syndrome |
| Small ears | Down syndrome |
| Low-set ears | Noonan syndrome, Down syndrome, Edwards syndrome |
| Hearing loss/deafness (infant – adolescent) | Apert syndrome, neurofibromatosis, Usher |
| **Syndrome** | |
| Hearing loss (child) | Alport syndrome, Fabry disease |
| Frequent ear infections | Turner syndrome |
| **Eyes** | |
| Structural defects of the eye | Alport syndrome, Homocystinuria, Horner syndrome, Keratoconus, Patau syndrome, Stickler syndrome |
| Staring/Excessive bleeding | Rett syndrome |
| Wide-spaced eyes | Down syndrome, Jackson-Weiss syndrome, Noonan syndrome, Apert syndrome, Coffin-Lowry syndrome, Wolf-Hirschhorn syndrome |

| Body system | Associated Genetic Disorder or Syndrome |
|---|---|
| Drooping eyelids | Horner syndrome, Apert syndrome |
| Epicanthal folds | Down syndrome |
| Down-slanted eyes | Coffin-Lowry syndrome |
| Up-slanted eyes | Down syndrome |
| Almond-shaped eyes | Prader-Willi syndrome |
| Lisch nodules of the iris | Neurofibromatosis |
| Absence of eye color in the iris | Aniridia |
| Cherry-red spot on the eye | Tay-Sachs, Neimann-Pick disease, Sandhoff disease |
| Cloudiness of the eye | Fabry disease, Stickler syndrome |
| Loss of visual acuity | Aniridia, Alport syndrome, Tay-Sachs disease, cone-rod dystrophy |
| Crossing of the eyes | Retinoblastoma |
| Retinal detachment | Ehlers-Danlos syndrome, Stickler syndrome |
| Cataracts (infant – adolescent) | Lowe syndrome, neurofibromatosis |
| Cat's-eye reflex | Retinoblastoma |
| Inability to distinguish color | Color blindness, cone-rod dystrophy |
| Glaucoma (infant – child) | Lowe syndrome, Aniridia, Stickler syndrome |
| Nystagmus | Leigh syndrome, Aniridia, spinocerebellar ataxia |
| Yellow sclera | Gilbert syndrome, Sickle cell disease |
| Photophobia | Anirida, cone-rod dystrophy |
| Doesn't like to make eye contact | Autism spectrum disorders |
| **Nose** | |
| Flattened nasal bridge or nose | Down syndrome, Robinow syndrome, Williams syndrome, Wolf-Hirschhorn syndrome |
| Beaked nose | Apert syndrome |
| Short nose with large tip | Coffin-Lowry syndrome |
| Impaired sense of smell | Kallmann syndrome |
| Frequent nosebleeds | Hemophilia, Factor V deficiency |
| **Mouth** | |
| Large or protruding tongue | Down syndrome |

| Body system | Associated Genetic Disorder or Syndrome |
|---|---|
| Tongue that is small | Stickler syndrome |
| Atrophy of tongue muscle | Spinocerebellar ataxia |
| High arched palate | Noonan syndrome |
| Cleft lip and/or cleft palate | Patau syndrome, Stickler syndrome |
| Wide or deep philtrum | Noonan syndrome |
| Short philtrum | Wolf-Hirschhorn syndrome |
| Flat philtrum | Fetal alcohol syndrome |
| Wide mouth with full lips | Angelman syndrome, Coffin-Lowry syndrome, Williams syndrome |
| Triangular-shaped mouth | Robinow syndrome, Prader-Willi syndrome |
| Delayed or absent speech | Angelman syndrome |
| Speech or swallowing difficulty | Angelman syndrome, spinocerebellar ataxia, Huntington's disease, Parkinson's disease |
| Expressive and receptive language delay | Autism spectrum disorders |
| **Teeth** | |
| Crowded teeth | Marfan syndrome, Noonan syndrome, Alpert syndrome |
| Wide-spaced or pointy teeth | Angelman syndrome, Coffin-Lowry syndrome |
| Dental abnormalities | Osteopetrosis, Ehlers-Danlos syndrome |
| **Skin/Hair** | |
| Café au lait macules | Neurofibromatosis |
| Xanthomas | Hypercholesterolemia |
| Angiokeratomas (dark red spots) | Fabry disease |
| Salty taste to skin | Cystic fibrosis |
| Light skin pigmentation | Albanism, Tuberous sclerosis |
| Telangiectasia | Ataxia-telangiectasia |
| Benign tumors on face | Tuberous sclerosis |
| Elastic-like or moveable skin | Ehlers-Danlos syndrome, Tuberous sclerosis |
| Thick skin | Hurler syndrome, Turner syndrome |
| Sparse, coarse hair | Menkes syndrome |

| Body system | Associated Genetic Disorder or Syndrome |
|---|---|
| Light color or white hair | Angelman syndrome, albanism |
| Easy bruising | Gaucher disease, Ehlers-Danlos syndrome, Factor V deficiency |
| Freckles in the groin or underarm | Neurofibromatosis |
| Jaundice | Galactosemia, Gilbert syndrome, sickle cell disease |
| **Hands/Feet** | |
| Single palmer crease | Down syndrome |
| Clenched hands | Patau syndrome |
| Long fingers | Marfan syndrome |
| Short fingers and toes | Down syndrome, Prader-Willi syndrome, Robinow syndrome |
| Curved fifth finger | Down syndrome |
| Clubbing of fingers | Pulmonary fibrosis |
| Finger contractions | Dupuytren contractures |
| Extra fingers or toes (polydactyly) | Patau syndrome, Smith-Lemli-Opitz syndrome |
| Hand or foot pain | Fabry disease, Lesch-Nyhan syndrome |
| Various foot abnormalities | Jackson-Weiss syndrome |
| Flat feet | Fragile X syndrome |
| Rocker-bottom feet | Edwards syndrome |
| High arches | Charcot-Marie-Tooth disease |
| Long arm span that exceeds height | Marfan syndrome |
| Fused fingers or toes | Apert syndrome |
| Curled toes | Charcot-Marie-Tooth disease |
| Hand flapping | Angelman syndrome, autism spectrum disorders, Rett syndrome |
| Hand tremor | Parkinson's disease |
| Peripheral neuropathy | Charcot-Marie-Tooth disease |
| **Heart** | |
| Structural defects | Williams syndrome, Marfan syndrome, Noonan syndrome, Patau syndrome, Turner syndrome |
| Aortic dilation | Marfan syndrome |
| Thickened heart wall | Hypertrophic cardiomyopathy, Danon disease, Pompe disease |

| Body system | Associated Genetic Disorder or Syndrome |
|---|---|
| Conductions defects | Long QT syndrome, Brugada syndrome, glycogen storage Disease, Wolff-Parkinson-White syndrome, short QT syndrome |
| Fainting episodes | Glycogen storage disease, hypertrophic cardiomyopathy, Wolff-Parkinson-White syndrome, short QT syndrome |
| High blood pressure | Polycystic kidney disease, familial hypercholesterolemia, Nneurofibromatosis |
| Palpitations | Wolff-Parkinson-White syndrome |
| Hypertension in a child | Familial hypercholesterolemia, Wilms Tumor, neuroblastoma |
| **Chest/Abdomen** | |
| Nipple placement that is wide or misaligned | Turner syndrome |
| Gynecomastia | Klinefelter syndrome |
| Depressed sternum | Marfan syndrome, Noonan syndrome |
| Small chest | Edwards syndrome |
| **Respiratory** | |
| Frequent upper respiratory infections | Cystic fibrosis, Neimann-Pick disease |
| Progressive shortness of breath | Pulmonary fibrosis, Leigh syndrome |
| **Gastrointestinal** | |
| Severe constipation/vomiting | Hirschsprung disease |
| Hepatomegaly or splenomegaly | Hemochromatosis, sickle cell disease, Hunter syndrome, Hurler syndrome, Gaucher disease, Pompe disease, Neimann-Pick disease, osteopetrosis |
| Liver failure | Galactosemia, hemochromatosis |
| Pancreatic failure | Hemochromatosis |
| Colon polyps at a young age | Lynch syndrome |
| **Renal system/ Genitourinary** | |
| Structural anomalies | Alport syndrome |
| Renal cysts | Polycystic kidney disease |
| Kidney stones | Lesch-Nyhan syndrome |
| Horseshoe-shaped kidney | Wilms tumor |

| Body system | Associated Genetic Disorder or Syndrome |
|---|---|
| Hematuria | Wilms tumor |
| Kidney disease or damage | Alport syndrome, Fabry disease, Bartter syndrome |
| Tumor | Wilms tumor, tuberous sclerosis |
| Sweet odor to urine | Maple Syrup Urine disease |
| **Muscular-Skeletal** | |
| Hypotonia (infancy) | Cri-du-chat syndrome, Down syndrome, Patau syndrome, Prader-Willi syndrome, Pompe disease, Krabbe disease, Leigh syndrome, Lowe syndrome, Menkes syndrome, Smith-Lemli-Opitz syndrome, Sandhoff disease, Wolf-Hirschhorn syndrome |
| Muscle atrophy | Muscular dystrophy, Charcot-Marie-Tooth disease |
| Abnormal flexibility of joints | Ehlers-Danlos syndrome, Fragile X, Marfan syndrome |
| Delayed walking | Muscular dystrophy, Angelman syndrome, Lowe syndrome |
| Psycho-motor regression | Neimann-Pick disease |
| Uncoordinated, jerky motor movement | Huntington's Disease, Lesch-Nyhan syndrome |
| Ataxia | Angelman syndrome, Leigh syndrome, fetal alcohol syndrome, spinocerebellar ataxia |
| Fragile bones | Osteogenesis imperfecta, Bartter syndrome, multiple myeloma |
| Paddle-shaped long bones | Pyle disease |
| Progressive muscle weakness | Muscular dystrophy |
| Short stature | Achondroplasia (dwarfism), hereditary multiple osteochondromas, Neimann-Pick disease, Noonan syndrome, Robinow syndrome, osteopetrosis, Prader-Willi syndrome |
| Bone pain | Ewing sarcoma, galactosemia, sickle cell disease, hemochromatosis, Pagets disease of the bone |
| Wide hips and narrow shoulders in a male | Klinefelter syndrome |
| Stiff limbs | Parkinson's disease |
| **Sex Organs/Hormonal** | |
| Underdeveloped or small sex organs | Klinefelter syndrome, Kallmann syndrome, Robinow syndrome |

| Body system | Associated Genetic Disorder or Syndrome |
|---|---|
| Delayed puberty | Kallmann syndrome, Klinefelter syndrome, Noonan syndrome |
| Infertility | Kallmann syndrome, Klinefelter syndrome, Noonan syndrome, Turner syndrome |
| Gynecomastia | Klinefelter syndrome, Klinefelter syndrome |
| Promiscuity | Huntington's disease |
| **Excessive laboratory values** | |
| High serum ferritin | Hemochromatosis |
| High cholesterol | Familial hypercholesterolemia, congenital nephritic syndrome |
| High bilirubin | Gilbert syndrome |
| Hypercalcemia | Williams syndrome |
| Increased serum ketones | Glycogen storage disease |
| Low red blood cells | Gaucher disease, sickle cell disease, multiple myeloma, Fanconi anemia |
| Low platelets | Galactosemia, Neimann-Pick disease |
| Excess amino acids in urine | Hartnup disease, homocystinuria |
| Proteinuria | Alport syndrome, congenital nephritic syndrome |
| Excess uric acid | Lesch-Nyhan syndrome |
| Hypercalciuria | Bartter syndrome |
| Excess salt in urine | Bartter syndrome |
| **Psychiatric** | |
| General personality changes | Huntington's disease |
| Aggression | Lesch-Nyhan syndrome, tuberous sclerosis |
| Gregarious or laughing personality | Angelman syndrome, Williams syndrome |
| Compulsive eating | Prader-Willi syndrome |
| Extreme interest in other people | Williams syndrome |
| Impaired social skills | Autism spectrum disorders, Klinefelter syndrome, tuberous sclerosis |
| Does not tolerate change in routine | Autism spectrum disorders, obsessive-compulsive disorder |
| Depression that lasts for weeks or longer | Major depressive disorder |

| Body system | Associated Genetic Disorder or Syndrome |
|---|---|
| Manic and depressive episodes | Bipolar disorder |
| Autistic-like behavior | Smith-Lemli-Opitz syndrome, Fragile X, tuberous sclerosis |
| Irritability/temper outbursts | Prader-Willi syndrome |
| Hallucinations | Parkinson's disease, schizophrenia |
| Exaggerated reaction when startled | Sandhoff disease |
| Delusions | Schizophrenia |
| **Aging** | |
| Premature aging | Progeria, early-onset Alzheimer's disease |
| **General** | |
| Failure to thrive | Galactosemia, Krabbe disease, Pompe disease, Leigh syndrome, Menkes syndrome, Neimann-Pick Disease |
| Lethargy | Galactosemia, hemochromotosis, Gitelman syndrome, sickle cell disease, Maple Syrup Urine disease, Fanconi anemia |
| High-pitched cat-like cry | Cri-du-chat syndrome |
| Irritability | Krabbe disease |
| Crave salt | Gitelman syndrome |
| Fascination with water | Angelman syndrome |
| Severe reaction to anesthesia | Malignant hyperthermia |
| Musty body odor | Phenylketonuria |

## CANCER RISK

Not all cancers are genetic, but when various types of cancer "run" in families, a genetic correlation should be expected. A three-generation detailed family history is valuable to this focused assessment. This is not an inclusive list of cancers that carry a genetic link. When there are multiple tumors (benign or malignant) during one's lifespan, the healthcare provided should suspect a genetic association (See Table 6.2).

Table 6.2

| Cancers With a Genetic Correlation: Multiple Tumor Locations | |
|---|---|
| Breast/bone/soft tissue/blood/adrenal glands | Li-Fraumeni syndrome |
| Colon/rectum/stomach/liver/endometrial | Lynch syndrome |
| Multiple bone tumors | Hereditary multiple osteochondromas |
| Adrenal gland/abdomen/chest/neck/pelvis | Neuroblastoma |
| Brain/blood/nerve sheath | Neurofibromatosis |

## CONCLUSION

Healthcare providers need to remain alert to the possibility of a genetic disorder to present anytime throughout the life cycle. Many complex genetic disorders and syndromes tend to reveal early symptoms during infancy and early childhood such as Down syndrome, Fragile X, Phenylketonuria. During childhood and adolescence, the risk for other genetic illnesses may be realized, such as cystic fibrosis, hypertrophic cardiomyopathy, or Marfan syndrome. As the individual progresses into adulthood, continued surveillance is necessary for early identification of genetic illnesses such as Lynch syndrome, Huntington disease, cancer, and early-onset Alzheimer disease.

It is important for the healthcare provider to continually consider a genetic association when assessment finding appear outside the expected norm, or if the symptoms is appearing in the less often affected sex, for example, male breast cancer. Additional screening and close monitoring for genetic disorders includes a detailed three-generation family medical history that identifies the medical history, cause of death, age of death, pregnancy and reproductive history (stillborn, miscarriage, spontaneous abortion), and environmental or occupational exposures (asbestos, lead, mold, agent orange). Ethnic risk for specific disorders should also be considered as part of the overall assessment.

## VIGNETTE

A 28-year-old male, Jake, presents to the physician complaining of constipation and some rectal bleeding. He works for a moving company and associated his symptoms with a poor diet and the possibility of hemorrhoids due to the heavy lifting that occurs on a regular basis. Prior to the examination the healthcare provider gathered a three-generation family health history and learned that other family members had been treated for "colon problems" and that his maternal grandmother died of cancer, but the patient was unable to clarify the type of cancer. Given the details ascertained from the family health history, the healthcare provider recommended a colonoscopy despite Jake's young age. The results of the colonoscopy showed multiple polyps. A biopsy was taken which confirmed the diagnosis of Lynch Syndrome. This is an autosomal dominant form of colorectal cancer. The early identification and subsequent treatment for Lynch Syndrome may have saved Jake's life. Knowing that an autosomal dominant inheritance pattern carries a 50% risk that it will be passed to offspring, Jake's siblings were screened for Lynch-syndrome which yielded two other family members with the disorder who will also begin treatment.

## REFERENCES

Jones, K. L., Jones, M. C., & del Campo, M. (2022). *Smith's recognizable patterns of human malformation*. Elsevier.

National Institutes of Health, National Center for Advancing Translational Sciences. (2022a). *FAQs about rare diseases*. Retrieved June 15, 2022, from https://rarediseases.info.nih.gov

National Institutes of Health, National Center for Advancing Translational Sciences, & Genetic and Rare Diseases Information Center. (2022b). *Find diseases by category*. Retrieved June 15, 2022, from https://rarediseases.info.nih.gov/diseases

National Library of Medicine, & Medline Plus. (2022). *Genetic conditions*. Retrieved June 15, 2022, from https://medlineplus.gov/genetics/condition/

# 7

# Environment and Genetic Impact

Dhaneesha Bahadur

*Our genetics are 99.9% similar, yet we are so very different. While some can eat all the packaged cupcakes from the local bodega and keep their glucose levels consistently within normal range, others are restricted to high-protein and high-fiber diets to keep diabetes at bay. Each of our health histories is unique, despite having only subtle genetic differences. One avenue to understand these differences is identifying how our genes interact with one another and how our exposures to different social experiences, lifestyles, and environments differ. Some have control of their environment, and others experience environmental risks and hazards that are difficult to manage and modify. Knowing one's genetic predisposition is only half of the battle: raising awareness of how the environment can increase one's risk of complex disease is the other.*

**In this chapter, you will learn:**

1. Types of environments and environmental risks that impact individuals genetically predisposed to complex disease
2. Gene–environment interaction and examples of diseases influenced by genes and the environment
3. The mechanisms of the epigenome and precision medicine
4. Health disparities and the environment

## Environment and Genetic Impact on Complex Disease

Genetics, genomics . . . synonyms, right? Wrong! Discussing the difference between genetics and genomics shines a light on *how* the environment can impact our genetics. Genetics refers to the study of genes and how certain traits and conditions are passed from one generation to the next. Genomics refers to the study of how these genes interact with one another AND with the person's environment. Genomics studies the complexity of diseases that are caused by a combination of genetic and environmental factors (National Institute of Health [NIH], National Human Genome Research Institute, 2020a). Researchers look to make sense of these modifiable and nonmodifiable variables to help individuals achieve an optimal level of health. Diabetes, cancer, heart disease, and asthma all are typically caused by both genetic and environmental factors. Healthcare workers can combine their knowledge of genetics and environmental risks to help improve health outcomes across one's life course by recognizing disease is based on this interchange of genes and environment. Institutions such as the Centers for Disease Control and Prevention (CDC) and NIH are working to discover how environment and genetics impact one another. With heightened national, and international, awareness, it is a disservice for nurses not to be aware of environment and genetic impact.

### *Defining the Environment*

Healthy environments are needed for optimal health, development, and longevity. From a healthy work environment to a healthy home environment, recognizing the importance of the surroundings in which one operates is essential. To build a healthy environment, the risk factors of said environment must be identified. The World Health Organization (2019) defines environmental risks as all the environmental physical, chemical, biological, and work-related factors external to a person, and all related behaviors.

**Essential Facts**

Examples of Environmental Risk Factors:

- **Physical:** Air Pollution, Extreme Temperatures
- **Chemical:** Pesticides, Lead, Asbestos
- **Biological:** Radiation, Viruses
- **Work-Related:** Coal Mining, Metal Mining

## Examples of Gene–Environment Interaction

Our exposure to environmental risks alone does not guarantee the diagnosis of disease. The experience leaves a mark on our genes that may cause changes to our phenotype, or the observable expression of our genotype. Different variants of genes, or genotypes, can cause different health outcomes when stimulated by environmental hazards or risks. This is a gene–environment interaction. Researchers have discovered there are many complex diseases that are examples of gene–environment interactions.

### *Autism Spectrum Disorder*

The word *autism* refers to a broad scope of developmental disabilities that impact a child's behavior, communication, and language. The causes of autism are believed by scientists to stem from genetics and the environment. Despite popular beliefs, celebrity opinions, and politics, the causes of autism must be supported with science rather than by unsupported claims. With recent media attention associated with autism, it is imperative to discuss peer-reviewed studies that offer scientific evidence of possible causes of autism. Nurses must be able to provide evidenced-based reasoning when questioned on causes of autism. Research identifying genotypes and environmental hazards can help reveal those at high risk for being diagnosed with autism, or autism spectrum disorder (ASD). The Childhood Autism Risks from Genetics and Environment Study is a population-based study that recruited preschoolers from California. The 251 participants were 24 to 60 months of age at the time of the experiment, had confirmed diagnoses of autism or ASD, and were exposed to air pollutants over the course of their lifetime. Residential histories were taken from the parent and included where the mother lived from beginning of conception to where the child currently lived (Volk et al., 2014). The results of the study reported subjects with the genotype *MET* rs1858830 and high air-pollutant exposure were at increased risk for autism as compared to subjects with the same genotype, but less ai-rpollutant exposure (Volk et al., 2014).

### *Parkinson's Disease*

Parkinson's disease (PD) is a neurodegenerative disorder that affects movement. Because PD is a progressive brain disorder, the symptoms start gradually and worsen over time. Clinical manifestations of PD may include difficulty walking, difficulty talking, memory difficulties, tremors, stiffness in the limbs and trunk, and fatigue. Neurons become impaired, or die, and lose their ability to produce normal levels of dopamine, which affects movement. Damage to nerve endings results in a loss of norepinephrine production. This causes changes in the sympathetic nervous systems, such as irregular heartbeat and sudden drops in blood pressure (NIH, National Institute on Aging, 2017). Although some cases of PD may be caused by genetic mutations, or may be hereditary, Parkinson's does not appear to run in families. Researchers believe PD to be caused by genetics and environmental risk factors, such as toxins. Paul et al. (2016) investigated the contributions of nitric oxide synthase (*NOS*) genes and organophosphate pesticides to PD risk, controlling for *PON1* (paraoxonase 1). The *PON1* gene increases the susceptibility of PD risk (Lee et al., 2013). The study included 357 participants who all had PD and were exposed widely to organophosphate pesticides from home and agricultural resources. Strong associations were found for PD in participants with *NOS1* genotypes exposed to organophosphate pesticides (Paul et al., 2016).

#### *Respiratory Syncytial Virus*

Respiratory syncytial virus (RSV) is a common respiratory virus, making it the most common cause of bronchiolitis and pneumonia in children younger than the age of 1 in the United States (Centers for Disease Control, n.d.). Up to 70% of children infected with RSV are diagnosed with bronchiolitis, but only 2% require hospitalization. RSV is the most frequent reason for infant hospitalization in the world, but causes of severe RSV bronchiolitis are still being researched (Caballero et al., 2015). In an Argentinian study of 418 patients with positive RSV, researchers explored the interaction between the *TLR4* genotype and the environmental exposure to lipopolysaccharide (LPS) (Caballero et al., 2015). The population selection criterion included healthy, term infants, and severity of RSV was determined by having an oxygenation status of less than 93%. LPS is a biological component of Gram-negative bacteria. Homes with low socioeconomic status had significantly higher levels of LPS when compared to homes with middle socioeconomic status. Infants living in lower socioeconomic status homes had direct exposure of LPS, evidenced by higher bedroom levels than those with higher socioeconomic statuses. Indirect exposure was evidenced by demographic indicators such as lack of sewage and crowding (Caballero et al., 2015). The presence of children with the *TLR4* genotype and who had exposure to biological environmental factors was significant, showing there is an interaction between genetics and environment in severe cases of RSV bronchiolitis (Caballero et al., 2015).

## Essential Facts

Genetics and environment both affect one's likelihood of being diagnosed with autism, PD, and respiratory syncytial virus (RSV).

## The Epigenome

Since the mapping of the Human Genome Project in 2003, science has been abuzz with new, exciting research. Genome mapping has revitalized epigenetics, the study of what is "above" or "on" the genome. Epigenetics is the branch of biology that addresses how genes are expressed. The term *epigenetics* was developed in the 1940s by Conrad Waddington when describing the interaction between genes and gene products, their role in directing development, and how they result in an organism's phenotype (Rogers & Fridovich-Keil, 2018). Through genomic medicine, epigenetics is understood in greater detail and is used to create personalized care. The epigenome is the interpretation of the chemical modifications associated with turning on and off gene expression. Research suggests it is the combination of the epigenome and environmental stimuli that create changes in our phenotypes.

Exposure to lifestyle and environmental factors causes pressures that illicit chemical responses to the genome, affecting the way DNA's instructions are used by cells. Epigenomics is the study of the multiple chemical compounds that instruct the genome what to do (National Human Genome Research Institute, 2020b). This instruction to alter gene expression can change over one's lifetime and can affect generations after.

## Essential Facts

"Epigenetics literally translates into just meaning 'above the genome.' So if you would think, for example, of the genome as being like a computer, the hardware of a computer, the epigenome would be like the software that tells the computer when to work, how to work, and how much."

*Source:* Jirtle, R. (2007). *Epigenetics (video clip)*. Retrieved September 30, 2021, from http://www.pbs.org/wgbh/nova/sciencenow/3411/02.html

## Environment and Social Determinants of Health

Healthy People 2030, updated from Healthy People 2020, reminds us health is an ever-evolving science that is meant to reflect the population's changing needs. The social determinants of health (SDOH) include economic stability, education access and quality, healthcare access and quality, neighborhood and built environment, and social and community context (U.S. Department of Health and Human Services, Office of Disease Prevention and Health Promotion, n.d.). In the United States many people live in areas that have unsafe air, unsafe water, and other health risks. There are four SDOH goals that include environmental health.

**Essential Facts**

1. Increase the proportion of people whose water supply meets Safe Drinking Water Act regulations – EH-03
   Target met or exceeded (Achieved target set at the beginning of the decade.)
2. Reduce the amount of toxic pollutants released into the environment – EH-06
   Target met or exceeded (Achieved target set at the beginning of the decade.)
3. Reduce the number of days people are exposed to unhealthy air – EH-01
   Baseline only (No data beyond the initial baseline data, progress unknown.)
4. Reduce health and environmental risks from hazardous sites – EH-05
   Baseline only (No data beyond the initial baseline data, progress unknown.)
   *Source:* Adapted from U.S. Department of Health and Human Services, Office of Disease Prevention and Health Promotion (n.d.). Retrieved September 30, 2021, from https://health.gov/healthypeople/objectives-and-data/social-determinants-health.

Physical environments defined in this chapter reflect tangible toxins and easily measurable hazards, such as unsafe water or air pollution. Living in neighborhoods that have disproportionately higher rates of violence than the national average is an example of a social environment that nursing professionals must consider when discussing environment and genetics. Low-income neighborhoods, racially profiled communities, immigrant populations, or refugee communities are all specific social environments that may impact one's genomes. Social factors contribute to our determinants of health through where people are born, live, learn, play, work, and age (U.S. Department of Health and Human Services, Office of Disease Prevention and Health Promotion, n.d.). SDOH are conditions in the environment that affect a wide range of health, functioning, and quality-of-life outcomes and risks (U.S. Department of Health and Human Services, Office of Disease Prevention and Health Promotion, n.d.). These social factors, exposure to lifestyle, and environmental factors cause pressures that illicit chemical responses to the genome, affecting the way DNA's instructions are used by cells. Epigenomics is the study of how these chemical responses instruct the genome what to do and how the instruction to alter gene expression can change over one's lifetime and can affect generations after (National Human Genome Research Institute, 2020b). Social environment and social experience affect gene function during various stages of life (National Institute of Health, National Cancer Institute, 2022). This is referred to as social epigenomics.

Understanding the environment-related SDOH can help address reasonable modifiable factors to make individuals healthy. Creating a safe environment for all is of utmost importance, but knowing there are populations at higher risk because of their genetics creates an even greater need to address environmental reform for the purposes of health promotion and reducing disparities.

## Environment and Health Disparities

Promoting healthy choices alone cannot eliminate health disparities. Multiple levels of community, government, and structural racism must be evaluated and reevaluated to better facilitate health equity for all. Vulnerable populations, such as people of color, have a higher risk of being unable to obtain the ideal SDOH. Deconstructing centuries of bias systems is an arduous task. Unfortunately, racial/ethnic minorities and people with low incomes are more likely to be exposed to harmful health and safety risks, contributing to further health disparities.

A pillar of being an effective healthcare professional is identifying vulnerable populations. In addressing vulnerable populations, we can identify health disparities and work to break down barriers that are obstacles to receiving quality healthcare. Merging the concepts of SDOH, environment, and genetic predisposition creates a platform for nurses to discuss the importance of being an advocate for health promotion within our communities.

## Essential Facts

Understanding diversity, equity, and inclusion is imperative when identifying vulnerable populations that are at higher risk for health

*(continued)*

*(continued)*

disparities. Environmental hazards and risk make gene expression more likely. Vulnerable populations are more likely to experience poorer living conditions that are unsafe and unhealthy.

## Environment and Precision Medicine

Genomic medicine is individualized care based on genomic information used for clinical care, health outcomes, and policy implications of that clinical use (National Human Genome Research Institute, 2020a). In 2011, there was a call to create a "new taxonomy" that defines disease not by physical signs and symptoms, but by underlying molecular and environmental causes (National Academy of Sciences, Engineering, and Medicine, 2011). Precision medicine, more specifically, is considered more accurate, patient centered, and multifaceted. Precision medicine utilizes genomics, epigenomics, environmental exposure, and other pieces of data to discover which interventions will be most beneficial for that individual (National Institute of Mental Health, 2011). Based on one's molecular structure and environment, individuals can be better prepared to face their health risks.

## Clinical Implications

Understanding genetics and genomics goes beyond the double helix one may imagine when thinking of this field of study. By keeping abreast of cutting-edge technology and recognizing the importance of the mapping of the human genome, nurses can use their positions as advocates to help promote healthy outcomes in the fight against complex disease. Translating the science from research to practice is in the hands of healthcare providers. Galvanizing nurses through education helps promote the dissemination of knowledge and promotes healthy lifestyles. Complex disease is multifactorial, creating the need for assessments that take into consideration environmental impacts. Using an interdisciplinary approach to nursing care promotes a holistic approach in achieving healthy populations. Recognition of diversity in our communities, support of health equity, and embracing inclusion are all avenues via which nurses can learn to protect the communities served.

Amid this interdisciplinary connectivity, it is imperative to remind nurses of theory and the totality paradigm: the person is a product of biological, psychological, social, and spiritual features

(Parse, 1987). These features are continually acting and reacting with the surrounding environment to accomplish goals and maintain balance. Present-day nursing is encouraged to view patients as a holistic being. Metaparadigms taught in nursing school stresses person, health, and environment. These metaparadigms are interconnected, and epigenomics gives evidence humans are a product of these metaparadigms. Although these metaparadigms are individual, they are fluid, one blending with the other to create Parse's concept of the human as being a result of biological, psychological, social, and spiritual features. Each feature can generate stress and directly affect gene expression. Not simply an empirical ideal, with molecular biology scientific evidence of these changes' being related to stressors can now be seen.

## CONCLUSION

Medicine, nursing, and genetic epidemiology are all disciplines studying the interaction between our genes and the environment. Using an interdisciplinary approach best elucidates how genes and environment interact. Nutritionists, biologists, nurses, physicians, researchers, and the general public read enthusiastically, trying to figure out how they can live longer, healthier lives. New information inspires new technologies, new ways of life. New information holds the possibility of generating new research. Each discipline helps in the creation and the dissemination of knowledge. Nurses can help *create* knowledge AND help *spread* knowledge to the populations we serve. Science is producing usable information that can change disease and how chronic conditions are viewed. From a nursing point of view, translation and communication of these advances are needed to make this information useful. No better profession exists to merge physical sciences and frontline healthcare services than nursing.

As the study of genetics grows and knowledge develops, we are able to enhance, transform, and elevate the level of care to populations we serve. Recognition of vulnerable populations can help us tap into avenues never ventured. Bridging biological science with nursing science is pregnant with possibility and is a necessity in bringing emerging research to the limelight. Epigenetics, social epigenomics, and precision medicine are concepts that are part of present-day healthcare. Epigenetics, for example, is the identification not only of high risk populations, but also of how the changes in gene expression can affect generations after (Weinhold, 2006).

## END-OF-CHAPTER QUESTIONS

1. Does the environment change your genetics?
2. What are examples of diseases that are impacted by genetics and environment?
3. How can understanding the epigenome and epigenetics help nurses in a clinical setting?

## REFERENCES


Caballero, M. T., Serra, M. E., Acosta, P. L., Marzec, J., Gibbons, L., Salim, M., Rodriguez, A., Reynaldi, A., Garcia, A., Bado, D., Buchholz, U. J., Hijano, D. R., Coviello, S., Newcomb, D., Bellabarba, M., Ferolla, F. M., Libster, R., Berenstein, A., Siniawaski, S., & Polack, F. P. (2015). TLR4 genotype and environmental LPS mediate RSV bronchiolitis through Th2 polarization. *Journal of Clinical Investigation, 125*(2), 571–582. https://doi.org/10.1172/JCI75183

Centers for Disease Control. (n.d.). *Respiratory syncytial virus infection (RSV).* Retrieved September 30, 2021, from https://www.cdc.gov/rsv/index.html

Jirtle, R. (2007). *Epigenetics (video clip).* Retrieved September 30, 2021, from http://www.pbs.org/wgbh/nova/sciencenow/3411/02.html

Lee, P. C., Rhodes, S. L., Sinsheimer, J. S., Bronstein, J., & Ritz, B. (2013). Functional paraoxonase 1 variants modify the risk of Parkinson's disease due to organophosphate exposure. *Environmental International 56,* 42–47. https://doi.org/10.1016/j.envint.2013.03.004

National Academy of Sciences, Engineering, and Medicine. (2011). *Toward precision medicine: Building a knowledge network for biomedical research and a new taxonomy of disease (2011).* Retrieved September 1, 2021, from http://dels.nas.edu/Report/Toward-Precision-Medicine-Building-Knowledge/13284

National Human Genome Research Institute. (2020a). *What is genomic medicine?* Retrieved September 1, 2021, from https://www.genome.gov/27552451/what-is-genomic-medicine/

National Human Genome Research Institute. (2020b). *Epigenomics fact sheet.* Retrieved September 1, 2021, from https://www.genome.gov/about-genomics/fact-sheets/Epigenomics-Fact-Sheet

National Institute of Health, National Cancer Institute. (2022). Epigenomics and epigenetics. Retrieved June 24, 2022, from https://epi.grants.cancer.gov/epigen/

National Institute of Health, National Institute on Aging. (2017). *Parkinson's disease.* Retrieved September 30, 2021, from https://www.nia.nih.gov/health/parkinsons-disease

National Institute of Mental Health. (2011). *Post by former NIMH director Thomas Insel: Improving diagnosis through precision medicine.* Retrieved December 2, 2018, from https://www.nimh.nih.gov/about/directors/

thomas-insel/blog/2011/improving-diagnosis-through-precision-medicine.shtml

Parse, R. R. (1987). *Nursing science major paradigms, theories, and critiques.* W.B. Saunders.

Paul, K. C., Sinsheimer, J. S., Rhodes, S. L., Cockburn, M., Bronstein, J., & Ritz, B. (2016). Organophosphate pesticide exposures, nitric oxide synthase gene variants, and gene-pesticide interactions in a case-control study of Parkinson's disease, California (USA). *Environmental Health Perspectives, 124*(5), 570–577. https://doi.org/10.1289/ehp.1408976

Rogers, K., & Fridovich-Keil, J. L. (2018). *Epigenetics. Encyclopedia Britannica.* Retrieved September 30, 2021, from https://www.britannica.com/science/epigenetics

U.S. Department of Health and Human Services, Office of Disease Prevention and Health Promotion. (n.d.). Retrieved September 30, 2021, from https://health.gov/healthypeople/objectives-and-data/social-determinants-health

Volk, H. E., Kerin, T., Lurmann, F., Hertz-Picciotto, I., McConnell, R., & Campbell, D. B., et al. (2014). Autism spectrum disorder: Interaction of air pollution with the MET receptor tyrosine kinase gene. *Epidemiology, 25*(1), 44–47. https://doi.org/10.1097/EDE.0000000000000030

Weinhold, B. (2006). Epigenetics: The science of change. *Environmental Health Perspectives, 114*(3), A160–A167.

World Health Organization. (2019). *Health, environment and climate change.* Retrieved September 5, 2021, from https://www.who.int/docs/default-source/climate-change/who-global-strategy-on-health-environment-and-climate-change-a72-15.pdf?sfvrsn=20e72548_2

# 8

# Ethics and Genetics

Michael J. Groves

*Genetics and ethics are as bound together as the DNA molecule itself. DNA is dynamic. It coils and uncoils, condenses, separates into chromosomes, and is nearly constantly active. So too for the ethics related to genetic science. Ethical considerations in genetics and genomics evolve in response to a rapidly growing science. Genetic science creates the potential to alter our health, appearance, and lifespan, and to redefine our human potential. Some of the essential questions raised by genetic technology include whether certain techniques should be used, how we can guarantee equitable global access to the benefits of genetic science, and how we can avoid or address the moral dilemmas associated with genetic and genomic science.*

**In this chapter, you will learn:**

1. Ethical theories and principles essential to addressing moral questions
2. Significant moral questions and dilemmas posed by advances in genetic/genomic science
3. An approach to discussing and potentially resolving these moral questions
4. An appreciation of the diversity, equity, and inclusion issues associated with this science

## ETHICAL THEORIES AND PRINCIPLES

Clinicians and bioethicists use several approaches to explore, understand, and resolve ethical issues related to healthcare, including genetic and genomic science. The nature of the ethical issue will determine whether a more broad theoretical approach should be taken, or a more focused case-based approach rooted in the application of ethical principles. It is helpful to have a sound understanding of the various theories and principles used to guide moral reasoning.

## ETHICAL THEORIES

Ethical theories generally fall into two main categories. Some are focused on what we do and are theories about our duties or theories of right action. These theories define our obligations to others or focus on what makes some actions moral and other actions not. Other theories are about who we are as people and are based in virtue ethics. These theories consider and define the characteristics that make someone a good or a bad person. Virtue ethics focuses on the development of our moral character and suggests that if we make ourselves more virtuous, then moral actions are more likely to follow. In this chapter we will focus on two theories of right action — deontology and consequentialism.

### Deontology

Deontology comes from the Greek words for duty (*deon*) and science or study (*ology*), and so deontology is the study of our duties and obligations to each other and to ourselves. Deontologists assert that morally correct actions are those that conform to some moral law or norm. The leading author of deontological theories is the German philosopher Immanuel Kant (1724–1804). According to Kant, morally worthy actions are those that are taken in response to a moral rule *and* are motivated only by a sense of duty. To define our duty, Kant uses what he called *imperatives.* He defined two types of imperatives: hypothetical and categorical.

Hypothetical imperatives include actions we should take if we want to achieve particular outcomes. If one of the talents we want to develop is to become an expert at playing the piano, hypothetical imperatives might include taking piano lessons and practicing the piano every day. We are not obligated to become a great pianist, but if we *want* to become one then we have a duty to do certain things.

A categorical imperative describes duties that must be honored without exception. Kant defines what he referred to as *the* categorical imperative, which he actually states in two different ways. The first formulation of the imperative states, "Act only on that maxim through which you can at the same time will that it should become a universal law" (Beauchamp & Childress, 2019). In this statement, Kant suggests that in order for an action to be considered moral, the action must be capable of being a universal law — that is, that everyone can do that action as they please. For example, if you are going to work under the maxim (rule) that it is okay to lie to a patient to get them to sign a consent form, then you must believe that it is acceptable for everyone to lie to patients for this reason. It should be clear that if we deceive patients to obtain consent from them, trust between nurses and patients would quickly break down and obtaining consent would ultimately be more difficult, not less. This deceit would also violate our obligation to respect the patient's right to autonomy and would violate the Code of Ethics for Nurses. Therefore, acting in such a manner would be inconsistent with our duty to the patient.

In his second formulation of the categorical imperative, Kant states, "Act in such a way that you always treat humanity, whether in your own person or in the person of any other, never simply as a means, but always at the same time as an end" (Beauchamp & Childress, 2019). This formulation demands that we treat everyone, including ourselves, not only as a means to an end, but also as an end themselves. What does it mean to be an "end"? Each of us possess unique goals, objectives, and desires that guide our lives and our actions. To treat someone as an "end" requires that we consider those goals and desires as we engage with people to achieve our own goals and objectives. Kant did not suggest that we cannot use other people to achieve our goals, only that we must consider their goals as well. For example, the registered nurse normally delegates work to the nursing assistant. For that delegation to be moral, the nurse must consider the needs of the nursing assistant as well. The nurse should assess what other work the assistant already has been assigned, whether or not the nursing assistant has had an appropriate break or mealtime, and if the delegation might keep the assistant from leaving on time at the end of the shift.

Kant's deontology ultimately leads to the consideration of all persons as having inherent worth and dignity. Rational adult persons are free to set the direction of their lives, determine their goals and objectives, and establish the rules by which they live. Creating rules that are aligned with the two formulations of the categorical imperative will keep people from interfering with the rights, goals, and ends of other persons and ensure we take actions that are considered in accord with the moral law. Next we consider the work of other theorists who contend that the correctness of actions is determined, not by moral laws and duties, but by the amount of "good" that those actions produce.

## Consequentialism

Unlike deontological theories that determine the morality of actions based on the action itself, consequentialist theories determine moral actions based on the outcome of those actions. Consequentialists believe that moral actions increase the "good" that people enjoy. What constitutes "the good" is subject to much debate. The good has been defined as happiness or the satisfaction of desires, and has been addressed in terms of both individual good and the more general welfare of society. Disagreements occur among consequentialists regarding the definition of the good, how it is measured, and whether the good should be equally divided among those concerned.

The primary consequentialist moral theory in bioethics is the theory of utilitarianism. Jeremy Bentham (1748–1832), and after him, John Stuart Mill (1806–1973), gave shape to the theory that would form a contrast to the duty-based obligations of deontology. Utilitarianism is a *consequentialist* ethical theory that defines moral actions as those that produce the most good. While morality for deontologists like Kant is centered in the action itself, for utilitarians like Bentham and Mill, morality is derived from the consequences of an action. If the outcome of an action is good, then the action is moral. While this is not a wholesale belief that the "ends justify the means," utilitarians believe that moral actions are those that produce the most good for the most people, all things considered.

Debates within the utilitarian school are about what constitutes "good." How is good measured? If I create a lot of good for one person, is that as moral as creating a little bit of good for many people? Bentham believed that good was defined simply as pleasure and that all pleasures were equal. The only determinant of the morality of an action was how much pleasure it created. Mill conversely defined a difference between higher and lower orders of happiness or pleasure. Baser pleasures such gluttony or desire were inherently less moral than more developed pleasures such as art, music, and literature.

One of the problems with the original formulation of utilitarianism was its requirement to maximize the good. This demand for maximization would theoretically permit harming some people so long as the good produced for others was greater than the harm imposed on some. The standard example used to demonstrate the excesses of this approach is the case of the transplant. In this scenario a surgeon has five patients, all of whom are about to die of organ failure. The surgeon also has one healthy patient who could serve as an organ donor for the other patients. A strict interpretation of utilitarianism would not only allow, but would require that the surgeon kill the healthy patient to save the lives of the other five. To overcome these excessive interpretations of consequentialism, theorists proposed three solutions. First, the idea of "satisficing" was offered as an alternative to maximizing. One only needs to produce enough good to satisfy the needs of others, not necessarily to maximize the good, thereby avoiding the excesses required by creating the most good possible. Second, consequentialists created a requirement that the creation of the good not make the situation worse for others by engaging in actions with negative outcomes. There is some discussion that these two approaches blur the lines between consequentialism and deontology. Finally, utilitarians made a distinction between act-utilitarianism and rule-utilitarianism. The original approach, act-utilitarianism, required the maximization of the good in each circumstance. The subsequent approach, rule-utilitarianism, distanced itself from maximization by inserting rules. In this approach, one only has to act in accordance with rules, which if generally followed, will produce the most good for the most people, all things considered. While both deontological and consequentialist theories are helpful in understanding the basis for moral action, they can be somewhat unwieldy in assisting patients and families in ethical decision-making. We now move to a consideration of the concept of principlism as developed by bioethicists Beauchamp and Childress.

### Essential Facts

Beauchamp and Childress have identified four principles that are particularly applicable to bioethics in healthcare: autonomy, beneficence, nonmaleficence, and justice. There is no established ranking or hierarchy of these principles. They should be considered to be of equal importance. It is also essential to realize that conflicts between two or more of these principles occur frequently in the context of healthcare decisions. Which principle should take precedence in any particular case will depend on the clinical situation and the moral questions under consideration.

### Principlism

The most commonly used approach in clinical bioethics, particularly in the tradition of the western world, is *principlism.* A particularly popular approach to principlism was developed by the bioethicists Beauchamp and Childress. In their work, they identify four primary principles of importance in healthcare situations:

- **Autonomy**: Literally meaning "self-governance," autonomy is the right of persons to make decisions about their lives and act in accordance with both their will and conscience.
- **Beneficence**: This principle speaks to our obligation to "do good." We are expected to act in the best interest of the patient and family.
- **Nonmaleficence**: This is usually discussed as the obligation to "do no harm." We are obligated to refrain from harming others and should take reasonable steps to reduce the potential for harm when possible.
- **Justice**: There are various "types" of justice. Social justice is concerned with the equitable distribution of burdens and privileges in a society, while distributive justice is associated with the distribution of resources. Resources can include food, water, housing, education, and access to healthcare, including genetic and genomic services.

## Autonomy

In healthcare, particularly in western cultures, there is a strong sense of duty to respect the right of patients to make their own decisions about their care. Generally, patients are free to consent to or refuse care and to choose among the available care options. Nurses both protect and respect the patient's autonomy by ensuring that patients have the capacity to make decisions and that, prior to providing care, we have the patient's informed consent to do so. Informed consent requires that the patient understand the risks, benefits, and alternatives among care options. The complexity of genetic information can present unique challenges to ensuring that patients understand the choices they have available to them.

## Beneficence

The principle of beneficence requires that nurses and other healthcare professionals act in the best interests of the patient. We also have some general obligations to beneficence, such as rescuing others who are in danger, when the risk to ourselves is small. There is, not infrequently, tension between our obligations to beneficence and to respecting the patient's autonomy. When the patient's autonomous choice is not in what we consider their own best interest, conflict can result. When patients make choices with which the healthcare team disagrees, there is often the potential to act paternalistically. Paternalism occurs when healthcare providers override the patient's autonomy in order to act in the patient's own best interest.

## Nonmaleficence

Often referred to as "the first principle" in medicine is the admonition to do no harm. We should refrain from any actions that cause unnecessary and avoidable harm to the patient and to mitigate the risk of harm to the best of our ability. Nonmaleficence is usually considered to be a more global requirement than beneficence. While it would be quite impractical to expect us to help everyone we encounter, it is not unreasonable to expect that we will refrain from causing harm to those we meet.

## Justice

While justice is a concept with which we are all familiar, it is a principle of incredible complexity and one that presents numerous challenges in making it a reality. In its most global sense, justice refers to equity and fairness. Of particular importance in genetics and genomics are both distributive justice and social justice. *Distributive justice* concerns the distribution of goods and services in a way that is fair. Inequities in the distribution of goods and services can result from a number of factors, such as excess demand, limited supplies, geographical issues, cost, and political issues. This principle represents a significant issue in genetic/genomic healthcare. Genetic testing, counseling, and treatment are both expensive and frequently not covered by insurance plans. Therefore, access to these services is often limited to those with the financial resources to pay directly. *Social justice* seeks equity in the distribution of privileges and burdens within society. Those working to ensure social justice in healthcare, and specifically in genetic/genomic services, seek to expose, understand, and eliminate discrimination and to ensure fair opportunity to enjoy the benefits of healthcare research and services.

In summary, the principles and theories discussed above do not represent divergent schools of thought that are disconnected and discontinuous. Adherence to these principles will generally work to maximize the good. Conversely, respect for autonomy and justice have a stronger connection to deontological theories and are usually directed at honoring our obligations or duties to others. These theories and principles are also clearly evident in the provisions of the Code of Ethics for Nurses (Fowler, 2015). For example, Provision 3 requires the nurse to advocate for and protect the patient's rights, clearly in line with respecting the patient's autonomy. The requirement in Provision 8 for the nurse to collaborate with others to protect human rights and reduce health disparities is a direct appeal to commit to engaging in social justice.

### Natural Law Considerations

Before moving on from this discussion of theories and principles, one more ethical theory should be presented. Natural law theory has been presented in both a religious and a secular context. In the religious context, natural law theory states that moral actions are those that are in accord with divine law, that obey God's will. Actions not in accord with the divine law are, by definition, immoral. In natural law's secular form, moral actions are those that conform to the natural functioning of the universe. This theory suggests that there is a natural way that the universe and its creatures are intended to act. When we act in those ways, then our actions are moral. While natural law is not generally used by bioethicists in determining right action, this theory does form the basis for the objections of some persons to the use of scientific and medical procedures, such as stem cell research and reproductive technologies (Vaughn, 2020).

## CONNECTING ETHICS AND GENETICS/GENOMICS

Having discussed several theories and principles of ethics, we now consider aspects of genetic and genomic sciences and healthcare that present unique challenges to our determination of ethical actions. The list of issues that follow will not sound very different from the usual list of ethical challenges in healthcare. When applied to genetic and genomic science, however, these ethical concerns can present additional complexities. While not a complete list of such challenges, below we introduce the ethics of privacy and confidentiality, genetic testing, the use of assistive reproductive technologies (ART), and finally consideration of the justice and equity issues in genetics/genomics.

### The Nature of Genetic/Genomic Data

What makes genetic and genomic data different from other sources of information about our patients? Genetic information provides a window into the current state and potential future for our patients and their families. For example, let us consider a patient being evaluated for type 2 diabetes mellitus (T2DM). This disease has both an environmental (lifestyle) component and a genetic component. The heritability, or incidence of the disease that can be attributed to genetics, ranges from 20% to 80% depending on the study (Ali, 2013). If we test this patient's blood glucose level we gain one piece of information about that particular patient at one specific point in time. If we test that same patient's HbA1C, we gain information concerning a longer period of time, but still only about that particular patient. If, however, we sequence the genes associated with T2DM or create a family pedigree focused on T2DM, we gain information about not only this particular patient, but also the entire family. Contained within our genetic code is information about not only ourselves, but also our entire family. When we diagnose one family member with a genetic disorder, we expose the potential risk of other family members for the same disease. The diagnosis of an autosomal recessive disorder in a child effectively diagnoses both parents as carriers of that disorder. Neither parent may have been aware of this status prior to the birth of their child. This diagnosis also identifies the parents' siblings and other blood relatives as potential carriers. One might consider that we are testing someone for the risk of a genetic disorder with neither their consent nor possibly even their knowledge. What steps are necessary to ensure that this information is used appropriately?

## Privacy and Confidentiality

From the preceding example it would appear that when genetics/genomics are concerned, our obligations to protect privacy and confidentiality may very well extend beyond our patient and include the patient's family. While privacy and confidentiality constitute ethical principles in their own right, they can also be considered under the principles of nonmaleficence and respect for autonomy. During the course of evaluation, diagnosis, and testing for genetic disorders or traits, a large amount of sensitive data is generated. In most organizations, this data is entered into and stored in electronic medical records. In many ways the privacy issues associated with genetic information are not necessarily all that different from issues surrounding other types of protected health information. These issues revolve around both access to information and the security of that information. For nurses, protecting patient and family confidentiality involves control of passwords, not leaving workstations unattended, not sharing passwords, and securing printed information. These obligations are not substantively different from the obligations to all patients.

The potential exists for privacy issues that might involve the breaking of the patient's confidentiality rather than its protection. When patients are diagnosed with genetic disorders that indicate substantial genetic risk for other family members and the patient refuses to disclose this diagnosis to others, consideration will need to be given to notifying family members against the wishes of the patient. The American Society of Human Genetics (1998) issued a statement defining the circumstances in which physicians and other professionals may be permitted to disclose genetic information to family members. Generally, if the patient will not disclose the information, the potential harm is serious, foreseeable, and highly likely to occur, the disease is preventable or treatable, and the benefit of disclosure outweighs the harm of doing so, disclosure by the appropriate professional should be considered. It may be helpful, when these issues arise, to seek consultation with the organization's ethics committee.

**Essential Facts**

Providers should consider disclosure of genetic information without patient consent when:

- Patient will not disclose the information
- The potential harm is serious, foreseeable, and highly likely to occur
- The disease is preventable or treatable
- Benefit of disclosure outweighs harm of doing so

## Genetic Testing

A wide range of techniques and processes fall under the topic of genetic testing. The types and purposes of genetic and genomic testing are covered in Chapter 11. The ethical issues related to genetic testing involve considerations of informed consent, the reporting of incidental findings, and the potential for misuse of test results. Within the broad topic of genetic testing, we will also consider issues related to direct-to-consumer testing (DCT).

Obtaining informed consent from patients is vital when genetic tests are performed, as with other tests and procedures. The collection of samples for genetic testing is usually quite simple, and involves collection of blood, tissue or hair samples, or saliva, or the taking of an oral or nasal swab. Results can take anywhere from a few days to several weeks, and patients should be prepared for the timing of results. Reference was made in the previous section to the disclosure of genetic test results to family members, potentially against the desires of the patient. This disclosure issue should ideally be addressed during the consenting process. The ordering provider should discuss the possibility of obtaining results that would be important to other family members. The provider and patient should decide, before the test is performed, how the disclosure to at-risk family members will be addressed. If the patient expresses reluctance to disclose results to family members, the reasons for this reluctance can be addressed and hopefully resolved before tests are performed.

Sometimes during genetic diagnostic testing, but perhaps more frequently during genetic research, incidental findings occur. In the research context an incidental finding is defined as a finding having potential health consequences for the research participant that is outside the scope of the study (Bevan et al., 2012). Incidental findings are also found in more conventional diagnostic situations. For example, a patient comes to the emergency department after a motor vehicle crash and has a chest x-ray done to rule out fractured ribs. On the radiograph the radiologist finds evidence of, as yet unknown, lung cancer. In this case, the ethical obligation to disclose this new diagnosis is clear. The potential harm from the cancer is obvious, and the patient should be informed about this finding. In genomic testing the situation is at times less clear. Incidental findings such as DNA mutations may be found, the significance of which is unknown. Ethical and clinical considerations in the disclosure of incidental findings include the pathogenicity of the finding, the likelihood of harm, the potential for treatment or prevention, the best interests of the patient, and the desire of the patient to have these findings disclosed.

A growing number of genetic tests are available to the general public that do not require authorization from a licensed provider. These direct-to-consumer (DTC) tests include genealogy tests offered by companies such as AncestryDNA and 23-and-Me. These companies offer products that trace the customer's genetic ancestry as well as provide testing for a variety of genetic traits and the markers for genetic disorders. DTC genetic tests are also available that assess carrier risk or test for the presence of certain risk alleles of a number of genes, such as the *BRCA1* and *BRCA2* genes.

Oversight for DTC genetic testing is conducted in the United States by the Food and Drug Administration (FDA). The FDA limits review of these tests to those for moderate- to high-risk medical purposes. Tests for nonmedical, general wellness or low-risk purposes are not reviewed by the FDA (U.S. Food and Drug Administration, 2019).

The ethics of DTC can be considered through the lens of beneficence. The developers and marketers of these tests propose that the tests provide a benefit to the consumer. To market these products ethically, the developer would need to ensure that the benefit experienced by the consumer outweighs any negative impact or potential harm the consumer may encounter. Harm might include anxiety or stress related to the results of testing, false negative or false positive results, or delays in results reporting. Generally we would consider the risk of genealogy-related tests to be low while we might consider the testing for risk alleles to be somewhat more anxiety producing. Steps that could be taken to reduce the potential for harm include clear explanations of the purposes of DTC testing, guidance for interpreting the results, and access in some cases to genetic counselors who can further explain results and provide referrals as appropriate.

**Essential Facts**

ART – Assisted reproductive technologies
IVF – In vitro fertilization
GIFT – Gamete intrafallopian transfer
PGD – Preimplantation genetic diagnosis

## Assisted Reproductive Technologies

Taken together, ARTs are a set of techniques and procedures designed to assist in procreation for individuals and couples who are unable to, or do not desire to, conceive and carry a pregnancy to term. Clients of these services include couples with fertility issues related to either ova or sperm; persons with physical obstructions involving the fallopian tubes, uterine issues, or cervical incompetence; single persons seeking parenthood; and same-sex couples requiring sperm or ova donors or the use of a surrogate to carry the pregnancy. ART includes artificial insemination, in vitro fertilization, gamete intrafallopian transfer (GIFT), preimplantation genetic diagnosis, sex-selection techniques, and others. Although this field continues to develop, artificial reproductive techniques have been in use since the 1970s.

Ethical considerations in the use of ARTs include issues of justice related to access to these services, questions regarding the use of healthcare dollars for these purposes, and objections to the use of these technologies based on natural law concerns.

Without doubt, ARTs are expensive. ARTs are also relatively "high-tech" and require a fairly sophisticated practice setting to ensure the safe use of these services. Additionally, these services are frequently not covered by traditional health insurance plans. In the United States, 15 states have laws requiring private insurers to cover some ART costs, and only eight states mandate coverage for ARTs.

Not only does this limited coverage affect access to these services, but also ART pregnancies in states without a coverage mandate were more likely to result in multiple births, preterm deliveries, and low-birth-weight infants (Centers for Disease Control and Prevention, 2016). Disparities in access and use of ARTs are also reported according to maternal race. In a 2021 analysis of 2017 data, researchers found a statistically significant association between maternal race and the use of ARTs (Ebeh & Jahanfar, 2021).

## Justice and Equity Issues in Genetics

In addition to the economic and racial disparities in access to genetic technologies, we can consider justice and equity issues related to concerns about misdirected ableism in the use of genetic technologies, and the representation of minority populations in genetic databases.

The combined use of in vitro fertilization with preimplantation genetic diagnosis allows for the selection of embryos that are free from the causative alleles for several disabling conditions. Some authors ask if the existence of these technologies creates an obligation on the part of parents to use them to avoid disability in an effort to provide the best possible life for their child? Williams (2017) suggests that three harms (to parents, other family members, and society in general) create a duty to avoid disability if possible. Inherent in the preceding question is an assumption that a life without disability is preferable to and of greater value than a life with disability. Some parents with what are considered disabilities reject this notion and opt for the opposite. In what some authors call "negative enhancement" parents choose traits such as deafness for their children to ensure entrance to a community to which the parents belong (Karpin, 2007). These issues raise questions about the very meaning of disability and the genetic obligations of parents to potential offspring.

The nature of genetic/genomic research often requires the use of large numbers of genomes from both public and private databases. The research conducted using these databases results in treatment recommendations and the development of new pharmaceuticals. To ensure that all persons secure the benefits of these scientific developments, these genomic databases would ideally include representation across a broad spectrum of the global population. Database administrators have struggled to add geographic diversity to these resources. These databases overrepresent people of European ancestry as compared to African, Asian, or Latin American populations. The relative lack of diversity in these databases results in limited genomic research that includes or is focused on these non-European peoples. Researchers found, for example, that in 413 genome-wide association studies on any type of cancer, only 4% of those studies involved underrepresented minorities, while 67% of studies were conducted on European populations (Landry et al., 2018). Genomic research would be enhanced by broadening the presence of diverse populations in genomic databases. The lack of such diversity perpetuates the presence of both ethical and medical disparities in genomic healthcare. One example of efforts of add to the diversity of genomic data is the *All of Us Research Project* sponsored by the U.S. National Institutes of Health. This program seeks to add genomic data as well as other healthcare information of at least one million people in an effort to further medical research.

The advancement of justice and equity in genomic research, education, and practice is an ongoing effort as it is in many other areas of healthcare and society in general. Nurses have a leading role in advocating for greater diversity in research, greater access to care, and greater opportunity in life.

## APPROACH TO ASSESSING MORAL DILEMMAS

There are a variety of models and approaches used to assist clinicians, ethicists, and patients and families in understanding and addressing moral conflict. One such model is presented here that is used quite commonly by ethics committees. The Four Topics approach is generally seen as a logical, organized way of approaching ethical issues and assists clinicians in considering all relevant factors in developing options. The model was developed by Jonson et al. (2015). Factors affecting ethical decisions are placed into four categories: Medical Indications, Patient Preferences, Quality of Life, and Contextual Features. Medical indications are associated with the principles of beneficence and nonmaleficence. Patient preferences consider issues related to respect for autonomy. Issues under quality of life concern beneficence, nonmaleficence, and respect for autonomy. Finally, contextual features generally consider issues related to justice and fairness. Often users of this model place the four topics into boxes, and so this model is referred to by come clinicians and ethicists as the Four Boxes Model (Table 8.1).

A full consideration of the issues and concerns associated with each of these features is beyond the scope of this text, but this model has been used extensively with success across a broad array of clinical ethics issues.

Table 8.1

**Patient Preferences**

| Medical Indications | Patient Preferences |
|---|---|
| Considers issues of beneficence and nonmaleficence<br>What is the patient's medical problem and what is the prognosis? | Considers issues of respect for autonomy<br>Is there informed consent for treatment? What are the patient's goals for treatment? Is the patient competent, and does the patient have decisional capacity? |
| **Quality of Life** | **Contextual Features** |
| Considers issues of beneficence, nonmaleficence, and respect for autonomy<br>What is the prognosis for a return to a "normal" life? | Considers issues of justice and fairness<br>Are there conflicts of interest with members of the healthcare team? What are the concerns and positions of family members? Are there issues of public health? |

## END-OF-CHAPTER QUESTIONS

1. Which of the following principles defines the obligation of the nurse to act in the patient's best interest?
   A. Justice
   B. Beneficence
   C. Nonmaleficence
   D. Respect for autonomy
2. "Negative enhancement" describes what action taken by parents?
   A. Use of preimplantation genetic diagnosis to prevent illness in their offspring
   B. Use of ART to ensure the best possible life for their child
   C. Intentional selection of embryos for implantation that pass disabilities onto their children
   D. Decision to forego having children to prevent disabilities
3. The categorical imperative is best described as which of the following?
   A. A moral law that must be followed in all circumstances
   B. A moral law that only applies to some circumstances
   C. The obligation to do the most good for the greatest number of people
   D. Respect for the patient's right to make their own choices
4. According to the secular statement of natural law, what is necessary for an action to be moral?
   A. The action must represent the free will of the person taking the action.

B. The action must be in accord with the natural functioning of the universe.
C. The action must be in accord with God's will for the universe.
D. The action must develop a natural ability of the person taking the action.

5. Which philosopher is most closely associated with deontological ethics?
A. Mill
B. Bentham
C. Aquinas
D. Kant

## REFERENCES

Alexander, L., & Moore, M. (2021). *Deontological ethics*. https://plato.stanford.edu/archives/sum2021/entries/ethics-deontological

Ali, O. (2013, August). Genetics of type 2 diabetes. *World Journal of Diabetes*, *4*(4), 114–123. https://doi.org/10.4239/wjd.v4.i4.114

American Society of Human Genetics. (1998). ASHG Statement: Professional disclosure of familial genetic information. *American Journal of Human Genetics*, *62*, 474–483.

Beauchamp, T. L., & Childress, J. F. (2019). *Principles of biomedical ethics* (8th ed.). Oxford University Press.

Berliner, J. L. (ed.). (2015). *Ethical dilemmas in genetics and genetic counseling*. Oxford University Press.

Bevan, J. L., Senn-Reeves, J. N., Inventor, B. R., Greiner, S. M., Mayer, K. M., Rivard, M. T., & Hamilton, R. J. (2012). Critical social theory approach to disclosure of genomic incidental findings. *Nursing Ethics*, *19*(6), 819–828. https://doi.org/10.1177/0969733011433924

Centers for Disease Control and Prevention. (2016, April 1). *ART and insurance*. Retrieved September 15, 2021, from https://www.cdc.gov/art/key-findings/insurance.html

Ebeh, D. N., & Jahanfar, S. (2021, March). Association between maternal race and the use of assisted reproductive technology in the USA. *SN Comprehensive Clinical Medicine*, *3*(5), 1106–1114. https://doi.org/10.1007/s42399-021-00853-z

Fowler, M. D. (2015). *Guide to the code of ethics for nurses with interpretive statements* (2nd ed.). American Nurses Association.

Jonson, A. R., Siegler, M., & Winslade, W. J. (2015). *Clinical ethics: A practical approach to ethical decisions in clinical medicine* (8th ed.). McGraw-Hill.

Karpin, I. (2007). Choosing disability: Preimplantation genetic diagnosis and negative enhancement. *Journal of Law and Medicine*, *15*(1), 89–102.

Landry, L. G., Ali, N., Williams, D. R., Rehm, H. L., & Bonham, V. L. (2018, May). Lack of diversity in genomic databases is a barrier to translating precision medicine research into practice. *Health Affairs*, *37*(5), 780–785. https://doi.org/10.1377/hlthaff.2017.1595

U.S. Food and Drug Administration. (2019, December 20). *Direct to consumer tests.* Retrieved September 27, 2021, from https://www.fda.gov/medical-devices/in-vitro-diagnostics/direct-consumer-tests

Vaughn, L. (2020). *Bioethics: Principles, issues, and cases* (4th ed.). Oxford University Press.

Williams, N. J. (2017). Harms to "others" and the selection against disability view. *Journal of Medicine and Philosophy, 42*, 154–183. https://doi.org/10.1093/jmp/jhw067

# 9

# Genetics and the Law

Nico Osier

*The overlap between genetics and the law is large and growing. There are laws that protect an individual's genetic information from getting obtained in certain unlawful ways, shared with the wrong individuals, and/or used to discriminate in certain contexts. Other laws protect individuals with disabilities associated with genetic disorders, set standards and funding for human embryo research, and restrict cloning. Beyond laws themselves, there was also a notable Supreme Court case about whether or not for-profit companies could patent genes. Additionally, there are numerous legal applications of genetic testing, including forensic analysis, paternity/maternity testing, and the use of embryos. The purpose of this chapter is to provide the reader with an overview of the key ways in which the law is relevant to genetics. It is important to note that this chapter was written by an author in the United States and does not reflect laws from other countries; readers located outside the United States are encouraged to explore the laws relevant to genetics in their home countries.*

**In this chapter, you will learn:**

1. The main laws related to genetics in the United States
2. The difference between lawful and unlawful acquisition of genetic information

3. The Supreme Court's ruling on gene patenting
4. Forensic and legal applications of genetic testing

## HEALTH INSURANCE PORTABILITY AND ACCOUNTABILITY ACT

Nurses and other healthcare providers are well versed in maintaining the confidentiality of protected health information (PHI) under the Health Insurance Portability and Accountability Act (HIPAA). However, many do not realize that there are some provisions in HIPAA that relate to genetics. Public law 104-109 (United States, 1996), better known as HIPAA, was first signed into law in 1996 and has since been amended. Increasingly, discussion became centered around how genetic information constitutes a special type of medical data, due in part to the fact that it requires a physician consultation and perhaps also counseling. Ultimately, this led to the addition of the HIPAA Security Rule in 1998 (H.R.3103; 45 CFR Part 160 and Subparts A and C of Part 164). Then in 2013, HIPAA was further amended to include the Omnibus rule, which expands upon the definition of "business associates" to include all companies involved in storing PHI and also states that genetic information is included in the definition of PHI (Goldstein & Pewen, 2013).

Specifically, PHI is covered under HIPAA if it is both (a) individually identifiable and (b) maintained by certain entities (e.g., healthcare provider, health plan, or healthcare clearinghouse). Some genetic information meets the criteria (denoted under (a) and (b) above) for PHI and is subsequently protected under HIPAA. For example, if a patient received genetic testing to diagnose, treat, or care for a known disease, the results of that genetic test would be covered under HIPAA because it is both considered identifiable and maintained by a healthcare provider. For additional information, see § 1320d–9, Application of HIPAA regulations to genetic information.

It is important to note that there are limitations in what is covered under HIPAA, because not all genetic information meets the definition of individually identifiable. A few examples of information that is not considered PHI, but rather research health information (RHI) and are thus not covered by HIPAA are provided here. First, aggregate genetic data that may be used as it is not individually identifiable. Occasionally diagnostic test results are done for research purposes that are not entered into the patient medical record; because these results are not maintained by a healthcare provider, they would not be covered under HIPAA. As a final example, HIPAA would not cover testing done in the absence of PHI identifiers as is sometimes done in exploratory genetic research for putative markers of disease or relevant promotor control elements.

## Essential Facts

- HIPAA covers PHI, which includes genetic information if it is individually identifiable and maintained by certain entities.
- HIPAA does not cover PHI including aggregate data, test results not linked to PHI, and/or testing not entered into the medical record.

## GENETIC INFORMATION NONDISCRIMINATION ACT

Genetic exceptionalism is the idea that genetic information is different from other PHI and, accordingly, requires additional protection beyond HIPAA. The next step in protecting genetic information was the Genetic Information Nondiscrimination Act (GINA), which was introduced in 1995 and signed into law (H.R. 1227/S. 306) in 2009 (United States, 2009). Since its original passage, GINA has been amended. Specifically, the Equal Employment Opportunity Commission (EEOC) wellness rules made it so that employers could no longer offer employees discounts on insurance premiums for participation in employer-sponsored wellness programs, since this was found to be in conflict with GINA as well as the Americans with Disabilities Act (ADA), discussed later.

Title I of GINA protects individual insurees from health discrimination in group health plan coverage by health insurers. This applies to both individual and group plans as well as to issuers of Medicare supplemental plans.

Title II of GINA protects applicants as well as current and past employees against discrimination on the part of employers, employment agencies, and labor organizations. Specifically, Title II protects against the unlawful acquisition, use, and disclosure of genetic information. Here, we will briefly break down what constitutes violations of this law.

Unlawful *acquisition* includes making direct requests for health-related information in a way that is likely to result in disclosure. Employers are also prohibited from requesting, requiring, or purchasing genetic information. It would also be considered unlawful acquisition to search an individual's personal effects, conduct internet searches likely to reveal genetic information, or actively listen in on third-party conversations. It is important to note that under

GINA the above mentioned actions would be considered unlawful whether there was intent to acquire the information or not. One company (Fabricut) was required to pay $50,000 in fees after it violated GINA by asking a new hire for her family medical history as part of the post-offer process and then violated the ADA by refusing to hire her due to her carpal tunnel syndrome (U.S. Equal Employment Opportunity Commission, Press Release 05-07-2013). Joy Mining Company was found to have unlawfully used their employees' data when they had new employees complete a preplacement form that requested family medical history information for certain conditions (U.S. Equal Employment Opportunity Commission, Press Release 01-07-2016).

Another main focus of Title II is protecting potential, current, and past employees from their employers' unlawfully *using* their information. It would be illegal to refuse or hire any applicant as a result of their genetic information; however, it is notable that this may be hard to prove in cases where there are multiple candidates with differing credentials and experiences. Title II of GINA also protects against employers' using genetic information to discharge employees based on their genetic information. Finally, GINA protects against employers' otherwise discriminating against applicants or employees with respect to the terms and conditions of employment. For example, an employer may not use genetic information to adversely affect applicant/employee status by limiting, segregating, or classifying employees based on their genetic information. The final element protected under Title II of GINA is that genetic information cannot be shared by employers except for in rare circumstances.

As was true for HIPAA, there are limitations to what types of genetic information are covered under GINA. There are specific types of information that are not covered under Title I or Title II of GINA. Notably, Title I of GINA only covers health insurance. There are, however, multiple other types of insurance, none of which are covered by GINA. For example, GINA does not protect against discrimination from other types of insurance including life, mortgage, car, motorcycle, renters, home owners, long-term care, and disability insurance. Notably, many of these types of insurance (e.g., long-term care; disability insurance) may be of critical importance to patients with genetic disorders; however, it is still lawful for these types of insurers to request genetic test results and use this information to make decisions about policy eligibility and pricing (Andrews, 2018).

Specifically, Title II of GINA only covers unlawful acquisition, use, or disclosure; however, there are several ways an employer could lawfully obtain or disclose genetic information. Lawful acquisition includes nonactively listening, but instead overhearing information.

It is also lawful if an employer finds out information through an employee's social media profiles; individuals are strongly recommended to not share their personal health and genetic information online. Likewise, finding out information about a person through publicly available documents such as newspapers is considered lawful. Other lawful acquisition includes obtaining information through a health or genetic service such as an employer-offered wellness program that is considered voluntary in nature, through a genetic monitoring program regarding biological effects of toxic substances in the workplace, through the Family Medical Leave Act (FMLA) or another related state-level leave certification process, or for law enforcement purposes. Lawful disclosure of genetic information is also possible. For example, under certain circumstances, when requested in writing, information can be disclosed to the employee/applicant themself or a family member. Disclosure to occupational health researchers for qualifying studies is also considered lawful. Finally, genetic information can be disclosed by employers for legal purposes, including in response to a court order, for use permitted by federal regulations, or to public health agencies at the local, state, or federal level in response to a public health emergency.

**Essential Facts**

- Title I of GINA prevents health insurers from discriminating against insurees.
- Title II prevents employers from unlawfully acquiring, using, or disclosing genetic information for their applicants, employees, and former employees.

## AMERICANS WITH DISABILITIES ACT

Public law 101-336, better known as the ADA, was proposed by the National Council on Disability in 1986 and passed in 1990 (United States, 1990). In 2008 the ADA Amendment Act (ADAAA), public law 110-325, was passed (United States, 2008). The ADA is a civil rights law that prohibits disability-based discrimination in various aspects of public life, including employment, access to government services/programs, and public transportation. ADA coverage includes physical/mental impairments that severely limit activities of daily life, records of such impairments, and being considered to have an impairment whether the perception is correct or incorrect. ADA does not include transient and minor impairments. It is also notable that the ADA only applies if someone already has a disabling condition, whereas someone with a genetic predisposition or disease, while not presently disabled, may still be a target of discrimination.

## OTHER LAWS RELATED TO GENETICS

Beyond the previously mentioned three laws (HIPAA, GINA, and ADA) there are a number of other laws that are relevant to genetic information. Some laws protect privacy in ways that supplement HIPAA and GINA or mandate standards for care. For example, the Medical Information Protection and Research Enactment Act of 2001 (H.R. 1215) protects patient privacy in a number of ways. First, it requires all health and research agencies to inform individuals regarding confidentiality procedures and to honor requests to view or amend their information if it meets certain criteria. It also prohibits such institutions from discussing PHI in the absence of written authorization or select other reasons. In addition, it outlines the consequences (e.g., civil penalties) for unlawful disclosure. The Prenatally Diagnosed Condition Awareness Act (H.R. 1353/S. 306) provides federal funding to support services for prenatally diagnosed conditions (e.g., Down syndrome); this law also provides guidelines regarding the education providers need to provide and the privacy of patient information.

Other laws surround the use of stem cells and/or embryos. For example, the Stem Cell Research Enactment Act of 2005 (H.R. 810) states that federal funds can be used for human embryonic stem cell research assuming certain conditions are met. To qualify, written informed consent must be obtained from the donors, who cannot be paid for the embryos, and the embryos must be destined for discarding if not used for research. The Joe Testaverde Adult Stem Cell Research Act of 2005 (H.R. 2541) provided federal funding to promote certain types of qualifying adult stem cell research via the establishment of centers for excellence. This law also directs the National Institutes of Health (NIH) to create a system for collection and preservation of relevant samples for stem cell research purposes. The Respect for Life Embryonic Stem Cell Act of 2005 (H.R. 2574) prohibits the creation of a human embryo from stem cells as well as derivation of stem cells from human embryos for clinical research purposes. In addition, this bill tasks the NIH with the creation of techniques for deriving stem cells without harming embryos and storing the resulting stem cells. Promotion of human stem cell research includes the Stem Cell Replenishment Act of 2005, which ensured at least 60 stem cell lines would remain available by revising the NIH guidelines to allow research on stem cells derived after August 2001.

Human cloning is addressed by federal law as well. The Right to Life Act of 2005 (H.R. 552) defines what it means to be a human being and includes human clones. A ban on human cloning in the United States is outlined in the Human Cloning Research Prohibition Act (H.R. 222). Further support for the ban on human cloning came from the Human Cloning Prohibition Act of 2005, which prohibits any person or entity involved in commerce from cloning (or attempting to clone) any human; in addition, this law prohibits efforts to receive or ship any human embryo created using cloning techniques.

## THE SUPREME COURT RULING ON GENE PATENTING

Scientists and the companies they work for want to protect their intellectual property and the ability to generate money from it. As a result, when the technology advanced such that we could learn about how certain DNA sequences impacted health, efforts to provide fee-for-service testing were under way. Consequently, more than 4,300 human genes were patented. Perhaps the most notable among them were the *BRCA1* and *BRCA2* genes implicated in some forms of hereditary breast and ovarian cancer, which was issued to Myriad Genetics (U.S. Patent 5747282). This positioned the company as a leader in the commercialization of genetic testing and earned them a lot of money. However, in 2013 *Association for Molecular Pathology v. Myriad Genetics, Inc.* reached the Supreme Court of the United States and forever changed commercialization of genetic testing. Specifically, the courts determined that DNA is a "product of nature" rather than a type of intellectual property that can be patented. Now that genes are not patented, companies can no longer hold exclusive rights to testing of genes (Association for Molecular Pathology v. Myriad Genetics, Inc, n.d.).

### Essential Facts

- According to the Supreme Court of the United States, genes are considered products of nature and cannot be patented.
- Myriad Genetics previously held a patent for *BRCA* mutation testing, but now that the gene is not patented, other companies can provide this service.

## DETERMINING FAMILIAL RELATIONSHIPS

A common application of DNA technology in legal cases is establishing familial relationships. Most commonly, this is in the form of paternity testing. In these cases, the mother's DNA is considered as a source of alleles and thus only informative alleles where the baby does not match the father are considered. More rarely, tests are done to determine maternity, as was the case in *Sarbah vs. Home Office, Ghana Immigration* of 1985 (Jobling, 2013). Other applications of DNA technology are determination of full and half-sibling relationships. Rationale for testing for familial relationships include child support cases, matching children to their families after detainment or natural disaster, as well as for identification of living relatives (e.g., siblings; grandparents).

**Essential Facts**

- DNA technologies are often used to establish familial relationships for the purposes of custody, child support, or reuniting families after a natural disaster or detainment.
- Most commonly paternity testing is done, but tests are also available for maternity testing and the establishment of other types of relationships (e.g., siblings; grandchild/grandparent).

## FORENSIC APPLICATIONS

Historically, solving crimes was dependent on detective work and eyewitness testimony. In the 1950s forensic analysis began to depend on hair analysis, which has flaws and is unable to uniquely identify a match, but rather can describe samples as "microscopically similar." Since then, hair analysis has been deemed flawed and proven to have led to many wrongful convictions (Norton et al., 2016). As techniques for analyzing DNA have become more available, the use of this technology in forensics has become more ubiquitous. Today, there are numerous forensic applications; a few key examples will be outlined here.

These technologies can be used to identify murder victims of unknown identity (i.e., solving a Jane/John Doe case). Depending on the state of decomposition of the body, the source of DNA may vary and could include tissue, hair with the root attached, bones, teeth, or blood. A match can be established using the suspected victim's personal effects (e.g., toothbrush) or by comparing to a living relative.

Another key application is that crimes can be solved by matching a suspect to a crime using genetic fingerprinting techniques. Often, these cases are solved by eliminating the victim's DNA as a source and considering all nonvictim DNA sources as possible suspects. Key sources of the suspect's DNA could include under the victim's fingernails, in the vagina/rectum (if a sexual assault occurred), or around bite marks. The crime scene should also be checked for sources of blood and saliva, including on things like soda cans and cigarette butts. It is important to keep in mind that there may be other reasons why an individual's DNA may be at a crime scene or even on a victim. For example, roommates, partners, and other intimate connections should be thoroughly interviewed and their alibis verified.

There are also forensic databases that are maintained and used to solve crimes that do not necessarily have suspects. The criteria for entry into these DNA databases vary by country and state. Likewise, the criteria for removal from the database vary and may be after a certain period of time, following release from prison, or dependent on acquittal. In some cases, suspects who are not proven to be guilty are entered into the database and never removed (Norrgard, 2008). In the United States, the National DNA Index System (NDIS) was established after being authorized by the DNA Identification Act of 1994 (H.R. 829/42 U.S.C. §14132). Subsequently, the criteria for entry into NDIS became mandated by law. The following categories of data may be maintained by NDIS: convicted offenders, arrestees, legal detainees, forensic casework, unidentified human remains, missing persons, and relatives of missing persons. This act also has requirements for participating laboratories relating to quality assurance, privacy, and expungement.

## END-OF-CHAPTER QUESTIONS

1. What must be true of genetic information in order for it to be covered under HIPAA?
   A. Personally identifiable information
   B. Research health information
   C. Maintained by a healthcare provider, health plan, or healthcare clearinghouse
   D. All of the above
   E. A and C only
2. Which of the following is covered under Title I of GINA?
   A. Long-term care insurers cannot discriminate against insurees on the basis of genetics.
   B. Disability insurers cannot discriminate against insurees on the basis of genetics.
   C. Health insurers cannot discriminate against insurees on the basis of genetics.
   D. All of the above
   E. A and C only

3. Which of the following is covered by Title II of GINA?
   A. Employers may not lawfully acquire, use, or disclose their employees' genetic information.
   B. Employees cannot discriminate against their employers based on their genetic information.
   C. Employers may not unlawfully acquire, use, or disclose their employees' genetic information.
   D. All of the above
   E. B and C only
4. Which of the following is/are a limitation of the ADA?
   A. It does not protect people with mental impairments.
   B. It does not protect people with short-term disabilities.
   C. It does not protect people with genetic mutations that increase their risk of future disability.
   D. All of the above
   E. B and C only
5. Which of the following is/are true about gene patenting?
   A. A 2013 Supreme Court ruling decided whether or not genes can be patented.
   B. Currently genes are considered to be products of nature and thus cannot be patented.
   C. Prior to 2013 genes were patented to protect commercial uses.
   D. All of the above
   E. B and C only

## REFERENCES

Andrews, M. (2018). *Genetic tests can hurt your chances of getting some types of insurance.* National Public Radio. https://www.npr.org/sections/health-shots/2018/08/07/636026264/genetic-tests-can-hurt-your-chances-of-getting-some-types-of-insurance

Association for Molecular Pathology v. Myriad Genetics, Inc. https://www.supremecourt.gov/opinions/12pdf/12-398_1b7d.pdf

Goldstein, M. M., & Pewen, W. F. (2013). The HIPAA Omnibus Rule: Implications for public health policy and practice. *Public Health Reports, 128*(6), 554–558. https://doi.org/10.1177/003335491312800615

Jobling, M. A. (2013). Curiosity in the genes: The DNA fingerprinting story. *Investigative Genetics, 4*, 20. https://doi.org/10.1186/2041-2223-4-20

Norrgard, K. (2008). Forensics, DNA fingerprinting, and CODIS. *Nature Education, 1*(1), 3.

Norton, J., Anderson, W. E., & Divine, G. (2016). Flawed forensics: Statistical failings of microscopic hair analysis. *Significance, 13*(2), 26–29. https://rss.onlinelibrary.wiley.com/doi/full/10.1111/j.1740-9713.2016.00897.x

United States. (1990). Americans with Disabilities Act [ADA] of 1990, Pub. L. No. 101-336. https://www.govinfo.gov/content/pkg/STATUTE-104/pdf/STATUTE-104-Pg327.pdf

United States. (1996). Health Insurance Portability and Accountability Act [HIPAA] of 1996, Pub. L. No. 104-191. https://www.govinfo.gov/content/pkg/PLAW-104publ191/pdf/PLAW-104publ191.pdf

United States. (2008). ADA Amendments Act [ADAAA] of 1990, Pub. L. No. 110-325. https://www.govinfo.gov/content/pkg/STATUTE-104/pdf/STATUTE-104-Pg327.pdf

United States. (2009). *The Genetic Information Nondiscrimination Act of 2008 (GINA).* Washington, D.C.: U.S. Department of Labor, Employee Benefits Security Administration.

U.S. Equal Employment Opportunity Commission, Press Release 05-07-2013. https://www.eeoc.gov/newsroom/fabricut-pay-50000-settle-eeoc-disability-and-genetic-information-discrimination-lawsuit

U.S. Equal Employment Opportunity Commission, Press Release 01-07-2016. https://www.eeoc.gov/newsroom/joy-mining-machinery-settles-eeoc-genetic-information-non-discrimination-act-lawsuit

U.S. Patent 5747282, Skolnick, H. S., Goldgar, D. E., Miki, Y., Swenson, J., Kamb, A., Harshman, K. D., Shattuck-Eidens, D. M., Tavtigian, S. V., Wiseman, R. W., Futreal, P. A., "17Q-linked breast and ovarian cancer susceptibility gene," issued 1998-05-05, assigned to Myriad Genetics, Inc., The United States of America as represented by the Secretary of Health and Human Services, and University of Utah Research Foundation. https://worldwide.espacenet.com/textdoc?DB=EPODOC&IDX=US5747282

# 10

# Genetic Screening

Christine Mladenka

*Genetic screening is defined as the process of testing asymptomatic individuals for pathogenic DNA variant(s) to identify those with an increased risk for having an inherited disease, developing a disease, and/or transmitting a disease to offspring (Andermann & Blancquaert, 2010; Burke et al., 2011; Hadley, n.d.). Four types of genetic screening will be presented, including carrier screening, noninvasive prenatal screening (NIPS), newborn screening, and cascade screening.*

**In this chapter, you will learn:**

1. The definition and purpose of genetic screening
2. Four different types of genetic screening, including carrier screening, noninvasive prenatal screening (NIPS), newborn screening, and cascade screening
3. The purpose, general process, and management of results for each genetic screening type

## GENETIC SCREENING

Genetic screening involves testing a population of asymptomatic individuals to identify those who have a pathogenic DNA variant(s) (also known as a mutation) that puts them at increased risk to have a particular genetic or inherited disease, develop a disease, and/or transmit a disease to offspring. For some genetic screening, those who test positive for a pathogenic DNA variant demonstrate an increased risk for disease associated with that variant. Individuals can undergo medical interventions to either reduce risk for being affected with the condition or to detect the disease early so treatment can be implemented to reduce the severity of the disease (Andermann & Blancquaert, 2010; Burke et al., 2011; Hadley, n.d.). Genetic screening is different than screening for other non-inherited conditions because it can also impact reproductive choices and can provide opportunities to decrease risk of having offspring with inherited conditions (Andermann & Blancquaert, 2010).

Genetic screening is optional and can occur across the lifespan (Raby et al., 2020). Carrier screening can be offered to adults preconceptually and prenatally. Targeted carrier screening and/or expanded carrier screening are supported by professional organizations (Raby et al., 2020). Carrier screening provides individuals/couples with information to consider when making reproductive decisions and to optimize pregnancy outcomes that align with their preferences and values (Edwards et al., 2015).

Prenatally, noninvasive prenatal screening (NIPS) is offered to determine fetal risk of having specific chromosomal abnormalities, such as Trisomy 21 (Down syndrome), Trisomy 13, Trisomy 18, and sex chromosomes. Results provide information to parents that helps them to make informed decisions about their pregnancy that align with their preferences and values (American College of Obstetricians and Gynecologists [ACOG], 2020).

Newborn screening is conducted on all infants born in the United States to determine if they are at increased risk for specific medical conditions that may jeopardize their health as a baby or child, despite appearing normal at birth. Necessary follow-up and medical management need to be implemented for positive test findings to reduce morbidity and mortality (Baby's First Test, 2021; Kemper, 2020).

Cascade screening is the process of notifying and informing adults of a biologic family member who tests positive for a pathogenic DNA variant for an inherited condition so that they are made aware of their potential increased risk. The relative is offered genetic counseling and testing, giving them the opportunity to make decisions regarding prophylactic interventions, as indicated, to reduce their risk for getting the condition, early interventions to manage the condition, and/or actions to avoid passing it onto offspring (National Cancer Institute, n.d.; Roberts et al., 2018).

## CARRIER SCREENING

Carrier screening involves testing adults for pathogenic DNA variants that may be passed onto offspring in an autosomal recessive (AR) or

X-linked inheritance pattern so that they can make informed decisions regarding reproduction that align with the individual's or couple's preferences and values (Burke et al., 2011). Traditionally, carrier screening for AR and X-linked conditions has been based on family history and for AR conditions prevalent in specific ethnic populations, such as Tay-Sachs disease in Ashkenazi Jewish population (ACOG, 2017b; Gregg et al., 2021; Raby et al., 2020). This has been referred to as targeted, or selective, carrier screening. Due to population intermixing in the United States leading to a diverse and multi-ethnic society, and to improved, less costly DNA analysis and sequencing, professional organizations also recommend offering expanded carrier screening to individuals who are pregnant or considering pregnancy (ACOG, 2017a; Edwards et al., 2015; Gregg et al., 2021).

Expanded carrier screening makes it possible to screen for a large number of inherited conditions simultaneously and without regard to race or ethnicity. Currently, conditions included on expanded carrier screening panels are determined by commercial laboratories with no defined standard or guideline; consequently, panels vary with the number of conditions screened, from ten to hundreds to thousands of disorders (ACOG, 2017a; Gregg et al., 2021; Rink, 2021).

Most conditions on panels are AR; however, a few panels include some X-linked and/or autosomal dominant single-gene disorders (Rink, 2021). Although information gained from expanded carrier screening can inform patient and provider shared decision making, it also presents practical challenges.

Professional organizations have developed guidelines regarding carrier screening for genetic conditions based on carrier frequency, prevalence, race or ethnicity, condition severity, and residual risk (Edwards et al., 2015). Key collective recommendations that professional organizations support include the following (ACOG, 2017a, 2017b; Edwards et al., 2015; Gregg et al., 2021):

- Offer carrier screening for cystic fibrosis and spinal muscular atrophy, plus specific inherited conditions as noted in an individual's personal and family history, to all individuals who are pregnant or considering pregnancy. Preconception carrier screening is preferred.
- Determine the best approach to carrier testing, sequential or concurrent screening.
    - Sequential testing involves carrier testing one individual, usually the female, and if positive results occur, testing the biologic father for the pathogenic DNA variant for the condition of concern. This will determine risk for affected offspring.

- Concurrent testing involves testing both individuals in the couple at the same time. This approach might be more appropriate for prenatal testing because prenatal diagnostic testing can be offered and conducted in a more time-efficient manner if both members of the couple test positive as carriers concurrently.

- Expanded carrier screening panels for adult-onset conditions is *not* recommended.
- Rescreening is not typically recommended unless the individual's medical history or family history changes.
- Carrier screening does not replace newborn screening.
- Provide pretest counseling:
  - Explain that carrier screening, both selective and expanded, is optional. The individual may decide to decline screening.
  - If screening during pregnancy, discuss screening and diagnostic test options available.
  - Use nonjudgmental and objective language to broadly explain the conditions screened on chosen panel, their inheritance pattern, phenotype, and prevalence.
  - Discuss risks, benefits, and limitations of screening, including unanticipated findings, such as variant(s) of undetermined significance.
  - Discuss that a negative result on screening test does not mean the fetus is not affected and does not guarantee a healthy child. Explain residual risk (chance that an individual is a carrier for other DNA variants not screened after a negative screening test).
  - Discuss that a positive result on prenatal screening test does not mean the fetus is affected. Further testing, including carrier testing of the biologic father, and prenatal and postnatal diagnostic testing, would be necessary to make a definitive diagnosis for the fetus.
  - Discuss cost of carrier screening and recommend that the individual check with their insurer on coverage.
- Provide posttest counseling:
  - Use nonjudgmental and neutral language to review results.
  - For negative findings, discuss how further evaluation is not currently indicated; however, residual risk for negative or low-risk test results is possible.
  - For positive or high-risk test results, discuss and provide written information that includes the following:
    - Information about the condition, including inheritance pattern, phenotype, and management strategies.
    - For AR conditions, the biologic father needs to be tested if not done so.

  - If one individual in the couple tests negative, no further actions are indicated as the risk for offspring to be affected is extremely low.
- Discuss reproductive options:
  - If both parents are identified as carriers of an AR condition, genetic counseling is indicated to help the carrier couple understand the increased risk that their baby may be affected.
  - If screening is preconceptual, genetic counseling should also include reproduction options to reduce or avoid risk of having an affected child. Options include:
    - They can choose to get pregnant, naturally, and undergo prenatal diagnostic testing.
    - They can choose to use in-vitro fertilization using egg or sperm donation and/or preimplantation genetic diagnosis.
    - They can choose not to have biologic children.
  - If screening is prenatal, counseling should also include options regarding diagnostic prenatal testing through chorionic villi sampling (CVS) or amniocentesis that allows for genetic testing of the fetus for the specific pathogenic DNA variant(s) associated with the AR condition. If the fetus tests positive for the DNA variant(s), the couple is counseled on options to continue the pregnancy and prepare to care for an affected child or terminate the pregnancy.
- Discuss potential implications for other biologic family members

Other guidelines regarding conditions included on expanded carrier screening panels differ among professional societies. The American College of Medical Genetics and Genomics (ACMG) presents a four-tiered approach that is consistent and ethnic and population neutral to promote equity and inclusion (Gregg et al., 2021). Tier 1 carrier screening, which includes carrier screening for cystic fibrosis, spinal muscular ataxia, and risk assessment, agrees with current ACOG (2017a) recommendations; however, ACMG recommends Tier 2 and 3 screening for all individuals who are pregnant or considering pregnancy, for a total of 97 inherited conditions. Tier 2 includes Tier 1 conditions plus selected inherited conditions with a ≥1/100 carrier frequency, such as sickle cell anemia, phenylketonuria (PKU), and usher syndrome, type A. Tier 3 includes Tier 2 conditions plus specific inherited conditions with a ≥1/200 carrier frequency, such as Joubert 9, and certain X-linked conditions, such as Fragile X and hemophilia A and B. Tier 4 carrier screening is appropriate in cases of consanguinity and as family or personal medical history warrants (Gregg et al., 2021).

ACOG (2017a, 2017b) recommends offering carrier screening to all individuals who are pregnant or considering pregnancy for cystic fibrosis and spinal muscular atrophy, plus specific conditions based on an individual's personal and family history and specific ethnicity (notably Eastern and Central European Jewish descent), and complete blood count and screening for hemoglobinopathies. ACOG (2017a) supports offering expanded carrier screening for genetic conditions with a carrier frequency of at least 1/100, with the caveat that conditions have well-defined signs and symptoms, have damaging effect on quality of life, require medical or surgical intervention, cause physical or mental impairment, or have early onset in life. Moreover, screened conditions diagnosed prenatally should have clinical opportunities to improve perinatal and infant outcomes. ACOG recommends clinical practices develop their own expanded carrier screening panels based on inherited conditions they determine best meet ACOG recommendations for their practice. For more details regarding professional organization recommendations for expanded carrier screening, please read references.

## NONINVASIVE PRENATAL SCREENING

NIPS (also referred to as noninvasive prenatal testing [NIPT]) is a prenatal screening offered to pregnant individuals as early as 10 weeks gestation to determine if their fetus has an increased risk for three chromosomal disorders: Trisomy 21 (Down syndrome), Trisomy 13 (Patau syndrome), and Trisomy 18 (Edwards syndrome). It is the most sensitive and specific prenatal screening option for these disorders (ACOG, 2020; Gregg et al., 2016). Professional organizations do not currently recommend NIPS for single-gene disorders or other autosomal chromosomal abnormalities (ACOG, 2020; Gregg et al., 2016). NIPS may be used to screen for sex chromosomal abnormalities; however, pretest counseling is recommended so patients understand exactly what the test is screening for, its limitations, and that it should not be used for biologic sex determination (Gregg et al., 2016).

NIPS involves analyzing a sample of maternal blood for fragments of cell-free DNA (cfDNA) from the fetus, which is derived primarily from placental trophoblasts released into the maternal blood stream from cells undergoing programmed cell death. The fetal component in maternal blood is known as the fetal fraction and makes up approximately 3% to 13% of the total cfDNA in maternal blood.

The quantity of fetal fraction must be at least 4% to avoid test failure (ACOG, 2020; Palomaki et al., 2021). Many factors can affect fetal fraction, including early gestational age, high maternal body mass index (BMI), inadequate sample collection, maternal use of heparin prior to 20 weeks, abnormal chromosome number, fetal or maternal mosaicism, and a pregnancy with more than one fetus (ACOG, 2020; Palomaki et al., 2021). Nine to 10 weeks gestation is generally the earliest to test as fetal fraction is usually high enough for successful testing and remains high throughout gestation; consequently, NIPS can occur any time after 10 weeks gestation. Studies demonstrate that pregnant individuals who weigh more than 180 to 250 pounds are at higher risk of having low fetal fraction even at 9 to 10 weeks gestation (ACOG, 2020; Gregg et al., 2016; Palomaki et al., 2021). Pregnancies with Trisomy 13 and 18 and Turner syndrome are also associated with low fetal fraction. Appropriate sample collection and preparation are important to preserve the fetal fraction in the blood sample (Palomaki et al., 2021).

## Essential Facts

It is paramount that staff follow laboratory directions for sample collection and preparation to prevent test failure.

Professional recommendations have been published by ACOG and ACMG. ACOG (2020) states that NIPS is an optional test that is routinely offered to pregnant individuals. ACMG states individual's preferences and values should play an important role in guiding the use of NIPS (Gregg et al., 2016). The importance of pre- and post-test counseling for individuals who are considering NIPS is emphasized by both professional organizations. Prior to testing, counseling should include the purpose of the screening and what it involves, possible results of the screening (positive, negative, and no call) and their implications, residual risk (risk of having an inherited condition that was not screened), and possibility of incidental findings that affect the individual, such as medical conditions reflecting an abnormality in her chromosome(s), mosaicism, or malignancy. If the individual chooses fetal sex determination, detection of an abnormal sex chromosome from the fetus or the pregnant individual is a potential finding (ACOG, 2020; Gregg et al., 2016). ACOG (2020) recommends a baseline ultrasound prior to NIPS to detect findings that may impact accuracy of results. These include an earlier-than-expected gestational age, viability of the fetus, number of fetuses, presence of a twin that is no longer viable, and fetal anomalies. Moreover, use of NIPS to test for other chromosomal abnormalities, such as microdeletions and genome-wide cfDNA testing for large deletions and duplication, is available through some laboratories; however, this screening lacks clinical validation and is not currently recommended (ACOG, 2020).

## Screen Results

Results from NIPS are commonly reported as screen positive, screen negative, or no call or no result, which means the interpretation of the test could not be done (Palomaki et al., 2021). All laboratories should report the fetal fraction on result report (Gregg et al., 2016).

### *Screen Positive Results*

Screen positive result indicates the fetus has an increased risk for the chromosomal abnormality and medical condition discussed in the report. Patients should be counseled regarding their revised risk, given information about the condition, offered genetic counseling services if available, and offered a comprehensive ultrasound evaluation with an opportunity for diagnostic testing, such as CVS or amniocentesis to collect fetal cells, to confirm results with karyotype analysis (ACOG, 2020; Gregg et al., 2016; Palomaki et al., 2021). Critical decisions, such as termination of the pregnancy, should *never* be based on results of NIPS (ACOG, 2020). If the patient declines diagnostic testing, pregnancy management should be based on serial ultrasounds and patient preferences, as well as appropriate intrapartum preparation to care for a potentially affected newborn (ACOG, 2020; Palomaki et al., 2021).

NIPS is a screening test, and false positive results can occur; however, they are less common than with other prenatal screening options. A false positive result means the fetus does not have the chromosome abnormality or medical condition associated with it but the screening result indicates that the fetus does have it (Palomaki et al., 2021). Potential causes of false positive results include mosaicism, in which there are cells in the fetus, placenta, and/or patient that have abnormal chromosomes and others have normal chromosomes, a deceased twin, maternal chromosome duplication, maternal cancer, mother is a transplant recipient or recently received donor blood, technical issues, and chance (ACOG, 2020; Palomaki et al., 2021). Because these situations are complicated and uncommon, referral to genetic counseling and diagnostic testing should be offered (ACOG, 2020; Gregg et al., 2016).

### *Screen Negative Results*

Screen negative results indicate that a fetus is at reduced risk for abnormalities of chromosomes tested and further testing is not usually necessary.

False negative results can also occur, although this is less common than with other prenatal screening options. A false negative result means the fetus has the chromosome abnormality or medical condition associated with it but the test result indicates that the fetus does not have it (Palomaki et al., 2021). Possible causes of false negative results include low fetal fraction, maternal chromosome deletion, placental mosaicism, error in specimen labeling, and technical issues (ACOG, 2020; Palomaki et al., 2021).

It is extremely important that the provider fully explain the limitations of the screening test. Although negative results for these specific chromosomes indicate reduced risk, the negative result does *not* guarantee the fetus is free from the conditions screened, due to false negative result, or from other chromosome and genetic abnormalities and other non-inherited conditions not screened, known as residual risk (Gregg et al., 2016; Palomaki et al., 2021).

### *No Call, No Result, or Failed Test*

Approximately 1% to 5% of NIPS do not produce a result and are reported as no call or no result (Palomaki et al., 2021). Possible causes include low fetal fraction, maternal use of low molecular weight heparin, some fetal chromosome abnormalities, suboptimal specimen collection or processing, twin pregnancy, and in vitro fertilization (Palomaki et al., 2021). Maternal obesity increases risk for a failed test because it is associated with low fetal fraction (Gregg et al., 2016). With no call results, ACOG (2020) recommends the patient be informed that such results are associated with increased risk for chromosomal abnormality, be referred to genetic counseling, and be offered comprehensive ultrasound evaluation and diagnostic testing. ACMG recommends offering diagnostic testing if result is due to low fetal fraction and maternal blood drawn at an appropriate gestational age; in cases of high maternal obesity, consider other screening options for abnormal chromosomes. ACMG also recommends all laboratories include the reason for the no-call on the report (Gregg et al., 2016).

## NEWBORN SCREENING

Newborn screening is a state-operated public health screening program that involves testing all newborns in the United States for a variety of medical conditions in order to detect and treat affected infants early to reduce morbidity and mortality. These conditions include cystic fibrosis, hearing loss, critical congenital heart defects, endocrine disorders, such as primary congenital hypothyroidism, hemoglobinopathies, such as sickle cell anemia, inborn errors of metabolism, such as PKU, and immunodeficiency (Kemper, 2020; Sontag et al., 2020; U.S. Department of Health and Human Services, 2018).

**Essential Facts**

During 2015–2017, the overall prevalence of babies identified with one of the disorders was 34.0 per 10,000 live births, which translates into approximately 12,900 births estimated to be identified with a disorder each year in the United States through newborn screening (Sontag et al., 2020).

All 50 states, Puerto Rico, Guam, the U.S. Virgin Islands, and the District of Columbia provide and manage newborn screening for approximately four million infants each year (Sontag et al., 2020). The Secretary of the Department of Health and Human Services recommends that all states screen for 35 core conditions on the Recommended Uniform Screening Panel (RUSP) as part of their newborn screening program (U.S. Department of Health and Human Resources, 2018). Each state determines the conditions to be screened based on several factors, such as state laws, financial cost of screening, frequency of disorder in the state, and availability of follow-up and treatment (Baby's First Test, n.d.). Important information about each state's newborn screening program, including a list of specific disorders screened by the state, an overview of the state's program, opt-out option, support for families, and storage and use of the dried blood spot, is available on the Baby's First Test website (Baby's First Test, n.d.).

Thirty-three of the 35 disorders in newborn screening are tested through laboratory screening of dried blood-spot specimens, and two conditions, hearing loss and critical congenital heart defects, are detected through point-of-care screening at the birth center prior to discharge (Sontag et al., 2020). The dried blood-spot specimen is obtained from a newborn heel stick within 24 to 48 hours of birth, sent to a state-designated laboratory, and analyzed for biochemical and genetic markers of diseases through mass tandem spectrometry (Centers for Disease Control and Prevention, 2008). Most state programs require a healthcare professional be informed of results.

### Positive or Abnormal Results

Positive, abnormal, or out-of-range results do not mean the infant has a disorder; however, speedy follow-up with parents and the primary health provider for diagnostic testing to confirm or exclude results found on newborn screening is warranted (Baby' First Test, 2021; Kemper, 2020). The primary care provider needs to be prepared to educate parents on the implications of positive results and take responsibility to ensure the infant undergoes appropriate diagnostic testing until a diagnosis is confirmed or excluded. Referrals to specialists and treatment centers may be necessary to ensure essential medical management for the infant so as to minimize the effects of the identified disorder (Centers for Disease Control and Prevention, 2008; Kemper, 2020). If diagnostic testing excludes the diagnosis, the primary care provider needs to educate and support parents regarding false positive results, addressing their anxiety and explaining why false positive results occur with screening tests (Kemper, 2020).

### Negative Results

Negative results usually need no follow-up actions; however, false negative results can occur, and the infant's primary healthcare provider needs to consider this should symptoms or physical findings develop in the child later in life (Kemper, 2020). Residual risk also remains for conditions not screened per individual state panels.

## CASCADE SCREENING

Cascade screening is the process of contacting and offering genetic testing to at-risk biologic relatives of an individual who has an inherited condition or tests positive for a pathogenic DNA variant(s) associated with that condition (National Cancer Institute, n.d.). Cascade screening usually starts with first- and second-degree relatives. This process may be repeated throughout the family as more affected individuals or pathogenic variant carriers are identified (National Cancer Institute, n.d.).

The purpose of cascade screening is to inform biologic relatives of their potential increased risk for an inherited condition, offer genetic counseling and testing, identify those who also test positive for a pathogenic DNA variant(s), and provide evidence-based surveillance and medical interventions to reduce the burden of disease (Roberts et al., 2018).

There are many challenges to provide effective cascade screening. Studies demonstrate there is no standardized process put forth by professional medical organizations in the United States (Roberts et al., 2018). Barriers abound, including limited communication between family members, low knowledge regarding cascade screening among family members and healthcare providers, cost issues, geographic challenges to testing, and varied state laws regarding privacy and release of genetic test results (Roberts et al., 2018). The Centers for Disease Control and Prevention (2014) has designated three hereditary conditions as Tier 1 genomic conditions that include cascade screening in the Genomic Application Toolbox: familial hypercholesterolemia, hereditary breast and ovarian cancer syndrome, and Lynch syndrome (a genetic condition that increases risk for colorectal and other cancers). More efforts to conduct meaningful intervention research are necessary to optimize cascade screening in the United States.

## END-OF-CHAPTER QUESTIONS

1. What is genetic screening?
2. A 45-year-old woman has been diagnosed with breast cancer and tested positive for the *BRCA1* gene mutation. What type of genetic screening needs to be discussed with the patient? Explain why.
3. A 25-year-old pregnant woman is 10 weeks pregnant. She has chosen to have NIPS at this time. Her result is a screen negative result. Explain what this means as if you are talking to the patient.
4. A couple is considering getting pregnant and are interested in carrier screening. What is the current recommendation for preconception carrier screening for a couple of European descent with no known family history of genetic conditions?
5. What is the state-based public health screening program for all newborns in the United States? How many and what medical conditions are recommended to be screened?

## VIGNETTE

A 30-year-old pregnant person who is 6 weeks pregnant chooses to undergo expanded carrier screening. She denies family history of genetic conditions. She tests positive for a pathogenic DNA variant associated with an autosomal recessive condition. Her partner, the biologic father, undergoes carrier screening and tests positive for a pathogenic DNA variant for the same autosomal recessive condition. They receive professional genetic counseling that includes information about the condition, symptoms, and medical management.

They are counseled that since they are both carriers for the autosomal recessive condition, the chance that their baby has the condition is 25% (baby has the pathogenic DNA variants for the condition on both genes). The chance that their baby does not have the condition and is not a carrier is 25% (baby does not have the pathogenic DNA variants on either gene). The chance that their baby does not have the condition but is a carrier is 50% (baby has only one gene that has the pathogenic DNA variant, like the couple). Prenatal diagnostic testing options are presented and offered to the couple to determine if their baby has the condition. They are told they can decline diagnostic testing and further evaluation for the condition will be conducted after birth. After pretest counseling, informed consent regarding risks, benefits, and limitations of the procedure and diagnostic test results and given time to privately discuss their options while considering their personal values and preferences, the couple decides to undergo chorionic villus sampling at 9 weeks gestation. Their insurer covers the cost of procedure and DNA analysis of fetal cells only for the pathogenic DNA variant of concern. The CVS procedure goes as expected without complication. Two weeks after the procedure is performed, the couple receives posttest counseling. Their baby has only one gene that has the pathogenic DNA variant, and no pathogenic DNA variant for the condition was noted in the other gene. Consequently, their baby does not have this autosomal recessive condition, but is a carrier. Routine prenatal and newborn management are indicated. Newborn screening will be conducted on their baby per their state program.

## REFERENCES

American College of Obstetricians and Gynecologists. (2017a). Carrier screening in the age of genomic medicine. Committee Opinion No. 690. *Obstetrics & Gynecology, 129*, e35–40.

American College of Obstetricians and Gynecologists. (2017b). Carrier screening for genetic conditions. Committee Opinion No. 691. *Obstetrics & Gynecology, 129*, e41–55.

American College of Obstetricians and Gynecologists. (2020). Screening for fetal chromosomal abnormalities. ACOG Practice Bulletin No. 226. *Obstetrics & Gynecology, 136*(4), e48–69.

Andermann, A., & Blancquaert, I. (2010). Genetic screening: a primer for primary care. *Canadian Family Physician, 56*, 333–339.

Baby's First Test. (2021). *Newborn screening 101*. https://www.babysfirsttest.org/newborn-screening/screening-101

Baby's First Test. (n.d.). *Conditions screened by states*. https://www.babysfirsttest.org/newborn-screening/states

Burke, W., Tarini, B., Press, N. A., & Evans, J. P. (2011). Genetic screening. *Epidemiologic Reviews, 22*, 148–164. https://doi.org/10.1093/epirev/mxr008

Centers for Disease Control and Prevention. (2008, October). *Newborn screening laboratory bulletin*. https://www-cdc-gov.libpublic3.library.isu.edu/nbslabbulletin/pdf/NSLB_Bulletin.pdf

Centers for Disease Control and Prevention. (2014, March 6). *Tier 1 genomics applications and their importance to public health*. https://www.cdc.gov/genomics/implementation/toolkit/tier1.htm

Edwards, J. G., Feldman, G., Goldberg, J., Gregg, A. R., Norton, M. E., Rose, N. C., Schneider, A., Stoll, K., Wapner, R., & Watson, M. S. (2015). Expanded carrier screening in reproductive medicine—Points to consider. A joint statement of the American College of Medical Genetics and Genomics, American College of Obstetricians and Gynecologists, National Society of Genetic Counselors, Perinatal Quality Foundation, and Society for Maternal-Fetal Medicine. *Obstetrics & Gynecology, 125*(3), 653–662.

Gregg, A. R., Aarabi, M., Klugman, S., Leach, N. T., Bashford, M. T., Goldwaser, T., Chen, E., Sparks, T., Reddi, H. V., Rajikovic, A., Dungan, J. S., & ACMG Professional Practice and Guidelines Committee. (2021). Screening for autosomal recessive and X-linked conditions during pregnancy and preconception: A practice resource of the American College of Genetics and Genomics. *Genetics in Medicine, 23*(10), 1793–1806. https://doi.org/10.1038/s41436-021-02103-z

Gregg, A. R., Skotko, B. G., Benkendorf, J. L., Monoghan, K. G., Baja, K., Best, R. G., Klugman, S., & Watson, M. S. (2016). Noninvasive prenatal screening for fetal aneuploidy, 2016 update: A position statement of the American College of Medical Genetics and Genomics. *Genetics in Medicine, 18*(10), 1056–1065. https://doi.org/10.1038/gim.2016.97

Hadley, D. W. (n.d.). *Genetic screening*. National Human Genome Research Institute. https://www.genome.gov/genetics-glossary/Genetic-Screening

Kemper, A. R. (2020). *Newborn screening*. UpToDate. Retrieved August 29, 2021, from https://www-uptodate-com.libpublic3.library.isu.edu/contents/newborn-screening?source=bookmarks_widget

National Cancer Institute. (n.d.). *Cascade screening*. https://www.cancer.gov/publications/dictionaries/genetics-dictionary/def/cascade-screening

Palomaki, G. E., Messerlian, G. M., & Halliday, J. V. (2021). *Prenatal screening for common aneuploidies using cell-free DNA*. UpToDate. Retrieved August 29, 2021, from https://www-uptodate-com.libpublic3.library.isu.edu/contents/prenatal-screening-for-common-aneuploidies-using-cell-free-dna?source=bookmarks_widget

Raby, B. A., Kohlmann, W., & Hartzfeld, D. (2020). *Genetic testing*. UpToDate. Retrieved August 29, 2021, from https://www-uptodate-com.libpublic3.library.isu.edu/contents/genetic-testing?source=bookmarks_widget

Rink, B. D. (2021). *Expanded carrier screening in pregnant women and women planning pregnancy*. UpToDate. Retrieved September 18, 2021, from https://www-uptodate-com.libpublic3.library.isu.edu/contents/expanded-carrier-screening-in-pregnant-women-and-women-planning-pregnancy?search=preconception%20and%20prenatal%20carrier

%20screening&source=search_result&selectedTitle=1~150&usage_type=default&display_rank=1

Roberts, M. C., Dotson, W. D., DeVore, C. S., Bednar, E. M., Bowen, D. J., Ganiats, T. G., Green, R. F., Hurst, G. M., Philp, A. R., Ricker, C. N., Sturm, A. C., Trepanier, A. M., Williams, J. L., Zierhut, H. A., Wilemon, K. A., & Hampel, H. (2018). Delivery of cascade screening for hereditary conditions: A scoping review of the literature. *Health Affairs*, *37*(5), 801–808. https://doi.org/10.1377/hlthaff.2017.1630

Sontag, M. K., Yusuf, C., Grosse, S. D., Edelman, S., Miller, J. I., McKasson, S., Kellar-Guenther, Y., Gaffney, M., Hinton, C. F., Cuthbert, C., Singh, S., Ojodu, J., & Shapira, S. K. (2020, September 11). Infants with congenital disorders identified through newborn screening—United States, 2015–2017. *CDC MMWR*, *69*(36), 1265–1268. https://www-cdc-gov.libpublic3.library.isu.edu/mmwr/volumes/69/wr/mm6936a6.htm?s_cid=mm6936a6_w

U.S. Department of Health and Human Services. (2018, July). *Recommended uniform screening panel.* https://www.hrsa.gov/advisory-committees/heritable-disorders/rusp/index.html

# 11

# Genetic Testing

Ana Lilia Fletes Rayas and José de Jesus Lopez Jimenez

*The methodologies used in genetic tests are very diverse, allowing the analysis of chromosomes up to a single nucleotide base, which is an important tool in the clinical field for both the diagnosis and prognosis of some genetic and even multifactorial diseases. This chapter provides a basic understanding of the definition and classification of genetic tests, as well as the requirements for the implementation of a genetic test and its clinical utility.*

**In this chapter, you will learn:**

1. The definitinion and classification of genetic tests
2. Methodological strategies for molecular genetic diagnosis
3. Requirements for the implementation of a genetic test
4. Validation and clinical utility
5. The relationship between clinician and laboratory

## PRINCIPLES OF GENETIC TESTS

Genetic testing is performed by analyzing genetic material, such as DNA, RNA, chromosomes, or proteins that are associated with an inherited disease or genetic disorder; the principal classifications of diagnosis tests are the diagnostic test and the predictive test (Lagos & Poggi, 2010). Diagnostic tests support confirmation of a clinically suggested genetic disease, while predictive tests are based on asymptomatic diseases and genetic predisposition. The asymptomatic diseases help to identify a late-onset illness' individual risks, and genetic predisposition tests can reveal, if an individual is positive, whether they have a greater risk of suffering from a particular disease, but without it can be assured that they will present the disease, such as in families with ovarian and breast cancer (*BRCA1* and *BRCA2*) (Yashon & Cummings, 2018). In addition, genetic tests can be used in pharmacogenetics (drug effects), inborn errors of metabolism, and paternity and maternity tests (Petersen, 2000).

## Essential Facts

- Genetic testing identifies DNA and RNA samples
- Preimplantation genetic test could diagnose diseases prior to birth
- Precision medicine is associated with genetics testing

Genetics and genomics have progressed greatly in the past few years, and conditions, such as prenatal diagnosis, predictive genetic testing in oncology, and monogenic and polygenic diseases, have a broad knowledge of the genetic interactions, so genetic counselling is very important to the study subject and their family for both the short and long term, and the ethical aspects are paramount (Than & Papp, 2017).

Almost all human diseases are influenced by genetic variation. The relationship between sequence variation and disease predisposition provides a tool for identifying processes fundamental to disease pathogenesis and highlights strategies for prevention and treatment. During the last few decades, the map of disease genes was focused on rare, monogenic and syndromic diseases. The pedigree tree and different technology are used to identify linkages in multiplex pedigrees in a family or in many families (different populations) (Claussnitzer et al., 2020).

The genome-wide association studies (GWAS), in which millions of genetic variants across the genomes of many individuals are tested to identify genotype–phenotype associations, have revolutionized the field of complex disease genetics over the past decade (Tam et al., 2019). The various techniques used to identify monogenic and polygenic inheritance and even some complex diseases, including cancer, chronic degenerative diseases, and prenatal diagnoses, are the polymerase chain reaction, used to identify polymorphisms and mutations (with their variants PCR end point, PCR in real time, and

PCR-RFLPs, among others), FISH technique, comparative genomic hybridization, and sequencing, among others, and recently including bioinformatics for the analysis of multiple sequences and even identifying protein folding and their interactions, have allowed us to carry out diagnosis and better knowledge of complex diseases (Claussnitzer et al., 2020; Krebs et al., 2018; Tam et al., 2019).

### Essential Facts

- Classical cytogenetics and molecular cytogenetics can be identified in the evolution of the techniques used in genetics.
- Molecular biology techniques used in genetics can detect single-nucleotide mutations and even tandem repeats to diagnose, and some polymorphisms or mutations detected through these techniques are currently being used to predict the behavior of some diseases.

## THE PEDIGREE FAMILY TREE TOOL, PHENOTYPE AND GENOTYPE IN CLINICAL AND GENETIC COUNSELING

Family history contains important information about the past of a person, and therefore about their family. The main function of this tool is to support the diagnosis, contributing to the clinician's decisions and identifying risk in other family members. Therefore, the genealogical tree provides information about possible transmission patterns and possible health problems that may arise due to the risk posed by family members or the patient himself. The timely identification of a greater risk allows the health professional to take measures for changes in lifestyle and even the monitoring of the patient or family member (Chapelle, 2009; Yashon & Cummings, 2018).

The family medical history must include at least three generations or affiliates. Some of the basic questions for gathering information about the family are as follows:

1. General information such as names and dates of birth of parents and siblings, uncles, aunts, and grandparents (this order is followed by first-, second-, and third-degree relatives, due to genetic segregation)
2. The origins of the family or racial or ethnic background and whether there was migration
3. The state of health, diseases, and the ages at which they were diagnosed will be included, including whether a very specific examination was needed for their diagnosis

4. Ages and causes of death, treatments provided, and the time of evolution of the disease
5. The clinical outcome of the pregnancies of the patient and of the relatives with a genetic relationship, including whether they were miscarriages in a period of early pregnancy, or deaths, as well as the age of the pregnancy and whether any fertility treatment was performed
6. Start of menarche, use of contraceptives, and if there are additional hormonal disorders (Figures 11.1a and 11.1b) (Kirkpatrick & Rashkin, 2017). Diverse informatic software are used to realize the family tree. It is possible to identify whether the disease being investigated has a pattern of segregation (remember that they can be autosomal dominant or recessive) or is inheritance linked to the dominant or recessive X.

**Essential Facts**

- The genealogical trees are tools that allow one to identify whether a disease has a segregation in the family or even if it is a novo disease.
- The genealogical trees, in addition to being simple to carry out, can be carried out in one or more families and identify various phenomena.

## CLASSICAL AND MOLECULAR CYTOGENETICS GENETIC TEST

Cytogenetic and molecular genetic analysis of neoplastic disorders, chromosomic rearrangement in chromosome instability syndromes, is important for the diagnosis, prognosis, and risk stratification to aid in the selection of treatment intensity, the identification of patients' eligibility for targeted drugs, and/or the monitoring of response to treatment in oncology diseases (solid and liquid tumors). The interpretation and reporting of these data according to international standards is so important for diagnostic laboratories. Karyotype, Fluorescent In Situ Hybridization (FISH), micronucleus assay, and chromosomal microarray analysis (CMA) are performed by array comparative genomic hybridization (aCGH) are the most used techniques for cytogenetic studies, and their results should be described according to the International System for Human Cytogenetic Nomenclature (ISCN; previously named International System for Human Cytogenetic Nomenclature) (Levy & Wapner, 2018; Stevens-Kroef et al., 2017) (Figure 11.2).

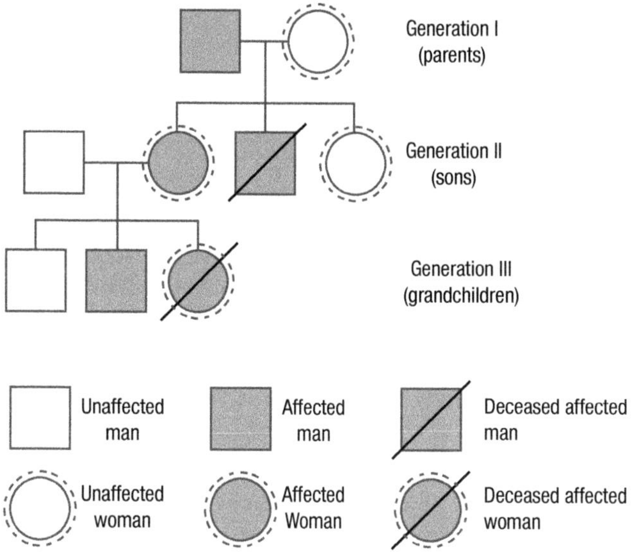


(A)

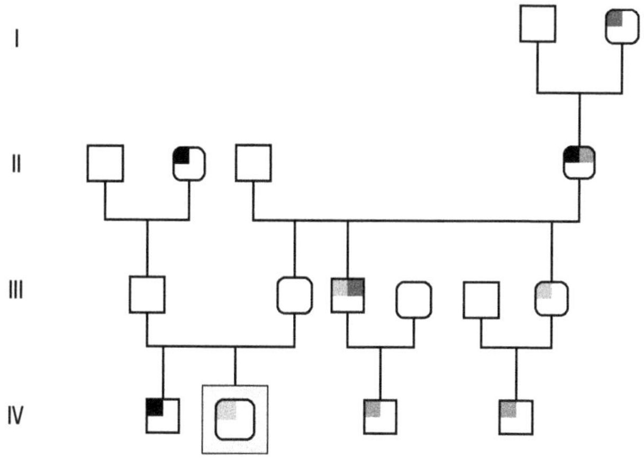


(B)

**Figure 11.1** **(A)** Family tree symbology for generations; **(B)** Pedigree of a family; generations available for study are indicated by Roman numerals I, II, III, IV; the clinical case is in shaded box (family tree of a patient currently in a study). The patient who comes to the consultation and who is under study is highlighted in shaded box, and light gray segment in the various generations represents the presence of breast cancer

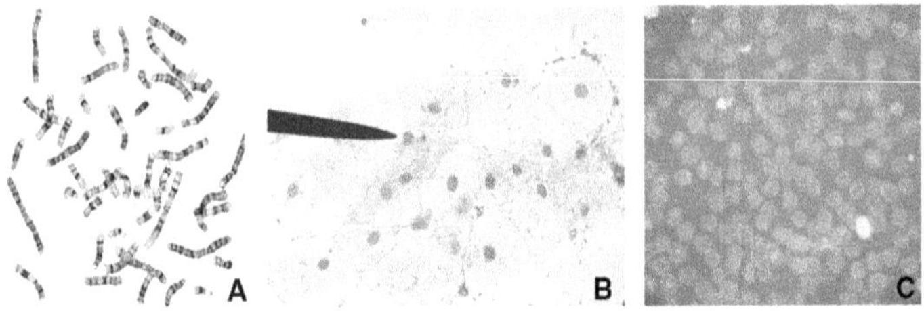


**Figure 11.2** Classical and molecular cytogenetic techniques for diagnosis and/or prognosis of genetic and chronic degenerative diseases
**(A)** Karyotype assay; **(B)** Micronuclei assay with Giemsa-Wright stain in bright field; **(C)** Micronuclei assay with an epifluorescence microscope with acridine orange.
*Source:* Images courtesy of Ana Lilia Fletes Rayas and José de Jesús López Jiménez

Recently, the micronucleus assay has been used in subjects who use pesticides and in chronic degenerative diseases due to its sensitivity in identifying chromosomal instability by environmental mechanism, such as genotoxicity and cytotoxic agents (López-Jiménez et al., 2020); it has also been reported that it could be used to biomonitor cytotoxicity in medication, such as antineoplastic drugs (Roussel et al., 2019).

- Classical and molecular cytogenetics tools continue to be used to detect some structural and numerical abnormalities in chromosomes.
- These techniques are usually complemented by molecular biology tools and the clinical association presented by the patient.

## MOLECULAR BIOLOGY TOOLS

Some molecular techniques have been combined with cytogenetic techniques (Table 11.1), such as in the case of fluorescence in situ hybridization (FISH), multiplexdependent ligation probe amplification (MLPA), and quantitative fluorescence-PCR (QF-PCR), which have been able to reduce the reporting of results to a period of 2 to 3 days. At the prenatal level, aneuploidies are the most common, as they have allowed the rapid detection (2 to 3 days) of the most common aneuploidies (Levy & Wapner, 2018; Mori et al., 2012).

Table 11.1

**Molecular Methodologies in Diseases**

| Assay | Methodology | Clinical Uses | Sensitivity | Test Specifications |
|---|---|---|---|---|
| **Conventional karyotype and their variante** | Karyotyping identifies numerical and structural changes in chromosomes | Identify structural abnormalities (i.e., translocations, inversions, large deletions, like so gains, and losses of complete chromosome sets) | Detect genomic abnormalities in megabases | Requires peripheral blood, mitotic and antimitotic agents are used, results are reported in several days. Some variants of conventional karyotype are Q, C (identify the heterochromatin of centromeric regions), G (giemsa staining is used), R (reverse), and Ag-NOR (identify the nuclear organization regions of the 13, 14, 15, 21, and 22 chromosomes) bands |
| **SCE (sister chromatid exchanges)** | Sister chromatid exchanges are used with bright field microscopy | Identify chromosomal instability; the increasing of the frequency of SCE indicates an increase in chromosomal instability | Low cost and requires an experiment be observed | To identify chromosomal instability, such as in chromosome instability syndromes |
| **FISH (fluorescent hybridization in situ)** | Identify small chromosomal abnormalities with fluorescent probes associated with complementary sequences of genetic material | Identify numerical and structural changes in chromosomes (i.e., amplifications, loses) is used in microdeletion syndromes and different leukemias) | Detect submicroscopic genomic rearrangements and has a high sensibility | Requires sequences of target chromosome for labeling; can be biased due to hybridization artifacts |

*(continued)*

Table 11.1

**Molecular Methodologies in Diseases (*continued*)**

| Assay | Methodology | Sensitivity | | Test Specifications |
|---|---|---|---|---|
| **CGH (comparative Ggnomic hybridization)** | It is based on marking the DNA of the propositus case with a green fluorochrome and comparing it with a normal or reference individual with a red fluorochrome and mixing them, performing an in-situ hybridization on normal chromosomes. | This test is a fast and accurate human genome study tool, by which DNA alterations, including microdeletions and duplications, can be detected. | High sensibility and sensitivity | Prenatal study of chromosomal abnormalities, which is responsible for evaluating the chromosomopathies in fetal DNA before birth and its association with a phenotypic spectrum and specific evolution |
| **Molecular Tools Used in Genetic Testing** | | | | |
| **PCR (polymerase chain reaction)** | Allows targeted amplification of template DNA or RNA with the addition of primers (forward and reverse) such as dNTPs and polymerases in an in vitro reaction | Broad clinical use, like identifying a rearrangement in a family tree, mutations, and polymorphisms associated with a disease | A single DNA or RNA strand may be enough to be amplified and could be from a blood or other sample tissue | Method may yield sequence errors during amplification of DNA, depending on polymerase fidelity |

| | | | | |
|---|---|---|---|---|
| **Sanger sequencing** | DNA sequencing technique using fluorescently labeled dideoxynucleotides to terminate a growing 3' DNA end selectively of a determinate fragment or organism | Identify somatic and germline mutations (point mutations) | Cannot detect mutant allele frequency <10%–20% | Limited sequencing length, short fragments of ~300–1000 base pairs |
| **RT-PCR (reverse transcription-polymerase chain reaction)** | Detection and amplification of a starting material of RNA by converting it to complementary DNA via reverse transcription | Is used for minimal residual disease monitoring of single-gene mutations and gene fusions/translocations | A single RNA strand can be amplified and is very sensitive | RT-PCR may be affected by genomic DNA contamination or another condition of the technique's initial RNA purity/fragmentation and is influenced by the types of primers used |
| **qPCR (quantitative polymerase chain reaction)** | Allows for the targeted amplification and real-time quantitation of DNA/RNA strands using fluorescent dyes | Used for mutational detection, gene rearrangements | Single DNA/RNA strand can be amplified and monitored in real time. Highly sensitive and accurate | Inadequate primer or probe design, degraded nucleic acid concentra- tion, improper standard curve can affect qPCR output |
| **"Droplet" digital PCR (polimerase chain reaction)** | Allows amplification of DNA/RNA by partitioning PCR reactions into water-oil emulsion droplets | Used for mutational analysis, liquid biopsy, and pathogen detection | Can detect individual strands of nucleic acid with a linearity over a range of 5 logs | Requires stable partitions to digitally separate reactions that may otherwise bias results |

*(continued)*

Table 11.1

| Molecular Methodologies in Diseases (*continued*) | | | | |
|---|---|---|---|---|
| **RNA-Seq** | Allows quantification and analysis of the transcriptome by converting the RNA strands to cDNA, followed by massively parallel sequencing using NGS platforms | Used for gene expression profiling, transcriptomic epigenetics, de novo transcriptome assembly, and variant calling for various clinical conditions | Current RNA sequencing kits can be used for gene expression from single cells that have approximately 10 pg of RNA material | Cost of sequencing may be higher compared to traditional gene expression methods like microarrays; depth of sequencing can affect the result; bias in readouts due to other sources of RNA based on abundance |
| **Single-cell sequencing** | Sequencing genetic material from a single cell by cell isolation, cell lysis, and library generation | Used to identify circulating tumor cell count, genetic heterogeneity, and mutations in cancer cells | Genetic material from a single cell can be sequenced | Technically challenging to isolate single cells; loss of genetic material during lysis; sparse DNA/RNA content |
| **Lumina sequencing (sequencing by synthesis)** | Method of massively parallel sequencing using fluorescently tagged nucleotides, which are sequentially added to DNA fragments adhered and captured on a solid surface. Sequencing by synthesis (SBS) | Used for DNA/RNA sequencing | Highly sensitive | Read lengths generally of 50–300 base pairs |

| | | | | |
|---|---|---|---|---|
| **Ion torrent (semiconductor based)** | Method of massively parallel sequencing using detection of a change in pH generated during normal DNA synthesis to determine which dNTP has been added | Used for DNA/RNA sequencing | High sensibility and sensitivity | Read lengths of 200 base pairs or more |
| **Cell-free DNA/ circulating tumor DNA/liquid biopsy** | Cell-free DNA (cfDNA) refers to DNA in blood that is not cell-bound. In the case of cancer patients, circulating tumor DNA (ctDNA) is the tumor component of cfDNA. Liquid biopsies could also represent cell-free RNA and DNA | Can be used to identify mutations in cancer when circulating tumor cells are not abundant. Can be used to monitor residual disease | Highly sensitive | Contamination from other samples may affect results. Typically coupled to NGS methodologies, and a high depth of sequencing is needed |

**Essential Facts**

Classical and molecular cytogenetics tools continue to be used to detect some structural and numerical abnormalities in chromosomes. These techniques are usually complemented by molecular biology tools and the clinical association presented by the patient.

## CONCLUSION

This chapter describes the clinical and laboratory techniques (classical and molecular cytogenetics) used in various hospitals where the diagnosis of genetic diseases is made or in those cases where the genetic load or the type of disease plays an important role in prognosis and treatment.

All genetic tests are used, and in some cases of classical or molecular kyogenetics, molecular biology techniques are added for the accurate diagnosis of the pathology. Therefore, the personnel who carry out genetic counseling for a patient must carry it out in the whole family by using genealogical trees to detect any pattern of allelic segregation.

Genetic tests that use molecular biology tools can be used in a single subject or in a population, which makes it possible to identify the Hardy–Weinberg equilibrium and thereby determine if there is a phenomenon in one's own family or in a community such as presence of inbreeding or a founder effect (Chapelle, 2009; Yashon & Cummings, 2018).

## VIGNETTE

Martha G. is a 26-year-old woman and a Guadalajara, Jalisco, native with a 5-year history of breast cancer. Martha has completed her chemotherapy treatment after a radical mastectomy of the right breast. There is no family history of breast cancer; however, there are chronic degenerative diseases such as diabetes mellitus, hypertension, and heart disease. A molecular panel is performed to detect mutations in the genes of *BRCA1* and *BRCA2*, and important clinical variants are found. When she arrives at the oncology service, a weight of 70.2 kg, 1.61 m height, and a BMI of 27.06 were identified. The tumor was detected by self-examination in the right breast of 7.5 cm, with a IIA clinical stage. Martha was diagnosed with an infiltrating ductal breast cancer, with negative progesterone receptors, negative estrogen receptors, and positive Her-Neu2. During the mastectomy procedure, 24 lymph nodes were removed and 25 cycles of adjuvant chemotherapy were applied.

- What will happen with Martha?
- Would her care be different if records were obtained immediately?

## REFERENCES


Chapelle, A. (2009). *Genetic Alliance; The New York-Mid-Atlantic Consortium for Genetic and Newborn Screening Services. Cómo entender la genética: Una guía para pacientes y profesionales médicos en la región de Nueva York y el Atlántico Medio.* Washington, D.C.: Genetic Alliance. https://www.ncbi.nlm.nih.gov/books/NBK132207/

Claussnitzer, M., Cho, J. H., Collins, R., Cox, N. J., Dermitzakis, E. T., Hurles, M. E., Kathiresan, S., Kenny, E. E., Lindgren, C. M., MacArthur, D. G., North, K. N., Plon, S. E., Rehm, H. L., Risch, N., Rotimi, C. N., Shendure, J., Soranzo, N., & McCarthy, M. I. (2020). A brief history of human disease genetics. *Nature, 577*(7789), 179–189. https://doi.org/10.1038/s41586-019-1879-7

Kirkpatrick, B. E., & Rashkin, M. D. (2017). Ancestry testing and the practice of genetic counseling. *Journal of Genetic Counseling, 26*(1), 6–20. https://doi.org/10.1007/s10897-016-0014-2

Krebs, J. E., Goldstein, E. S., & Kilpatrick, S. T. (2018). *Lewin's genes XII.* Jones & Bartlett Learning.

Lagos, L. M., & Poggi, M. H. (2010). Tests genéticos: Definición, métodos, validación y utilidad clínica. *Revista Médica de Chile, 138*(1). 128–132. https://doi.org/10.4067/S0034-98872010000100019

Levy, B., & Wapner, R. (2018). Prenatal diagnosis by chromosomal microarray analysis. *Fertility and Sterility, 109*(2), 201–212. https://doi.org/10.1016/j.fertnstert.2018.01.005

López-Jiménez, J. de, J., García-Ruvalcaba, A., Méndez-Magaña, A. C., Granados-Manzo, C. E., Rosales-Rivera, L. Y., García-Morales, E., Ayala-Buenrostro, P., De Alba-Espinoza, L. V., Ángel-del Río, A. C., Gaona-Sánchez, F., & Fletes-Rayas, A. L. (2020). Association of micronuclei frequency and other nuclear anomalies with flaxseed diet in metabolic syndrome patients. *Archives of Medical Science.* https://doi.org/10.5114/aoms.2020.96978

Mori, M. Á., Mansilla, E., García-Santiago, F., Vallespín, E., Palomares, M., Martín, R., Rodríguez, R., Martínez-Payo, C., Gil-Fournier, B., Ramiro, S., Lapunzina, P., & Nevado, J. (2012). Diagnóstico prenatal y array-hibridación genómica comparada (CGH) (I). Gestaciones de elevado riesgo. *Diagnóstico Prenatal, 23*(2), 34–48. https://doi.org/10.1016/j.diapre.2012.02.003

Petersen, G. M. (2000). Genetic testing. *Hematology/Oncology Clinics of North America, 14*(4), 939–952.

Roussel, C., Witt, K. L., Shaw, P. B., & Connor, T. H. (2019). Meta-analysis of chromosomal aberrations as a biomarker of exposure in healthcare workers occupationally exposed to antineoplastic drugs. *Mutation Research/Reviews in Mutation Research, 781*, 207–217. https://doi.org/10.1016/j.mrrev.2017.08.002

Stevens-Kroef, M., Simons, A., Rack, K., & Hastings, R. J. (2017). Cytogenetic nomenclature and reporting. Wan En, T. S. K. (Ed.), *Cancer cytogenetics* (Vol. 1541, pp. 303–309). Springer.

Tam, V., Patel, N., Turcotte, M., Bossé, Y., Paré, G., & Meyre, D. (2019). Benefits and limitations of genome-wide association studies. *Nature Reviews Genetics, 20*(8), 467–484. https://doi.org/10.1038/s41576-019-0127-1

Than, N. G., & Papp, Z. (2017). Ethical issues in genetic counseling. *Best Practice & Research Clinical Obstetrics & Gynaecology, 43*, 32–49. https://doi.org/10.1016/j.bpobgyn.2017.01.005

Yashon, R. K., & Cummings, M. (2018). *Genetic testing: What do we know?* Momentum Press, LLC.

# 12

# Population-Based Genetics

Kathryn N. Robinson

*This chapter will provide a thorough introduction to the field of population-based genetics as a central component of how variants and evolutionary forces influence evolutionary change over time, and the impact on genetic-related diseases at the population level. Goals of this chapter include understanding the importance of genetic variation diversity and how it provides key insights into the mechanisms of evolution. Numerous fields use genetic technology, including research, medicine, biotechnology, and engineering, to modify, enhance, add, or delete genes associated with certain genetic diseases in hopes of eliminating or preventing disease. Population-based genetics contributes to how we understand the influence of genetic information by identifying disease risk and susceptibility, leading to the integration of best practices for personalized medicine in disease prevention.*

**In this chapter, you will learn:**

1. The importance of population-based genetics in healthcare
2. The role of genetic variation in human population diversity
3. How evolutionary forces (mutations, genetic drift, migration, and selection) are mechanisms for evolutionary change that influence gene frequencies differently over time
4. Examples of genetic-related diseases in high-risk groups at the population level
5. How targeted genomic education affects healthcare-related decisions

## THE ROLE OF POPULATION-BASED GENETICS IN HEALTH

The availability of genetic information coupled with its integration in healthcare practice promotes a better understanding of disease etiology, intervention, and management. Population-based genetics is a fundamental component of policy, practice, and its role in public and community health. Population-based genetics is a subfield of genetics that deals with genetic differences within and between populations and is a part of evolutionary biology. When discussing health at the population level, genetics can help track and identify groups of individuals susceptible to developing certain health problems across generations. Genetics has become an influential component of understanding an individual's history and current health status as a biological determinant of health. This relationship between whether particular alleles or genotypes will become more or less common over time reflects the interaction between genetic variation, phenotypes, and environmental pressures. Studying population-based genetics provides important information concerning public health, including genetic determinants of pathogenicity and epidemiology, leading to enhanced management and development of innovative prevention strategies for complex diseases.

## POPULATION-BASED RESEARCH USING GENETICS

Population-based research can help us to identify variations in health and disease among people and across populations. There are several different ways to conduct population-based research using genetics. One way is to offer population-based genetic testing (PBGT), a method used for precision prevention that incorporates individual variation in genetic, epigenetic, and nongenetic (e.g., environment, hormonal, lifestyle, and behavioral) factors (Evans & Manchanda, 2020). Offering PBGT is an alternative strategy that helps individuals overcome limitations of clinical criteria/family-history-based genetic testing. This knowledge can help us identify the causes and effects of diseases, and find groups of people who are at increased risk, including those with hereditary variations that can be passed down through generations (Centers for Disease Control & Prevention [CDC], 2017).

A second way to conduct population-based research using genetics is with biobanks. Biobanks are large collections of biological and medical data and tissue samples (usually human) and have become a powerful tool in the study of complex diseases. These large repositories have become essential for improving personalized medical approaches, including effective use of biomarker identification (i.e., identify biology and detect presence of biological activities and processes), and are a critical step for disease diagnosis and prognosis (Coppola et al., 2019).

## Essential Facts

Population-based genetics:

- Is fundamental to understanding the composition of a population.
- Can help identify groups susceptible to a particular health problem.
- Uses biobanks and PBGT as two ways to conduct clinical research with genetic samples.

## HOW MUCH DO HUMAN POPULATIONS DIFFER?

The study of human genetic variation and its relationship to evolutionary history has led to scientific discovery with medical implications. These evolutionary histories are embedded in our genomes and can tell a significant story of what drives certain diseases within individuals and between populations. But what is genetic variation? Genetic variation refers to diversity in gene frequencies, which is how often (frequency) an allele occurs in a gene pool (population). Genetic variation can refer to differences between individuals and populations and contains useful information about population history and its relevance to medicine. Mutation is the ultimate source of genetic variation, but mechanisms such as sexual reproduction and genetic drift contribute to it as well (National Human Genome Research Institute [NHGRI], n.d.).

Population-based genetics has become a crucial element when exploring genetic variation diversity, which can inform personalized predictions about health status. The advancement of technology since the Human Genome Project has shaped how we measure genetic variation by allowing us to capture genetic marker data and allele frequencies, which leads to the ability to map the variation distribution between populations all around the world. Therefore, human genetic variation diversity influences disease risk and susceptibility and helps us infer aspects of human evolutionary history (Lu et al., 2014). As a result, personalized medicine has become an emerging practice that tailors medical treatment to an individual's characteristics by using biologic and genetic information of that individual to understand what makes them susceptible to disease and to guide decisions on how to best diagnose, manage, and treat that individual. According to Benton et al. (2021), "accounting for the innovations, adaptions and trade-offs that have shaped human populations, evolutionary histories and perspectives should be considered in the clinical application of precision medicine to complex disease" (p. 278).

A goal in identifying common and rare variants is to diagnose, treat, and forecast future disease risk. Rare variants are alternative forms of a gene that are present with a minor allele frequency (MAF) of less than 1.0%, meaning the genetic variants are only present in one or a few individuals. These rare variants enrich our understanding of important alleles as they relate to disease. Rare variants located in different genes could play a role in disease susceptibility and can now be captured by using approaches that use specific genetic variations with particular diseases, such as genome-wide association studies (GWAS). GWAS have proven successful in discovering common variants in numerous novel regions of the genome not suspected to have been involved with certain disease pathways (Saint Pierre & Genin, 2014). The purpose of using GWAS is to scan genetic markers across the genomes of many people to find genetic variations associated with a particular disease (NHGRI, 2020). The use of GWAS to associate specific genetic variations with particular diseases has been widely used in European, Hispanic or Latin American, Asian, and African populations.

**Essential Facts**

- Human genetic diversity is that any two humans differ, on average, in about 1 in 1,000 DNA base pairs (0.1%).
- Genetic variation refers to differences among the genomes of members of the same species.
- Identifying common and rare variants will help diagnose, treat, and forecast future disease risk in diverse populations.

## PATTERNS OF HUMAN GENETIC VARIATION

Human genetic diversity and evolutionary forces continue to shape patterns of variation across the genomes of diverse human populations. These variations are continuously influenced by biologic and environmental circumstances that cause fluctuations and adaptations over time. There are four major evolutionary forces: mutations, genetic drift, migration, and selection, all of which are mechanisms for evolutionary change that influence gene frequencies differently through time.

- **Single-base-pair differences**: This is considered the most common genetic polymorphism (differences). This type of polymorphism is called *single-nucleotide polymorphism (SNP).* SNP technologies have been successful in identifying disease-causing genes in humans, especially an individual's susceptibility to drugs, environmental toxins, and disease risk. These variations occur at a rate of 1 in every 100 to 300 nucleotides in the human genome and are responsible for 90% of genetic variation between humans (Cargill et al., 1999).
- **Mutations**: Mutations are a common method by which new alleles develop in a gene pool. These changes in the sequences of genes in DNA are one source of genetic variation. The mutation rate in humans continues to fluctuate depending on the type of mutation. However, the average human mutation rate is $1.0–1.5 \times 10–8$ per bp per generation, including ~30 new DNA variants with each gamete (The 1000 Genomes Project, 2011). The frequency of mutations in SNPs is relatively high since it is considered a polymorphism as compared to other types of gene mutations. Mutations create an avenue for genetic variation to occur, which acts as an evolutionary force that fuels variability in populations, thus enabling evolutionary change.
- **Migration and genetic drift**: Migration is the movement of genetic diversity (such as gametes) within a species. Genetic drift is considered a type of migration and describes at-random fluctuations in the distribution of genes in a given generation that differs from the distribution in the previous generation. This change occurs in the frequency of an allele within a population over time, which can lead to large changes within a population over a short period of time. A notable example of genetic drift is Gaucher disease among individuals of Ashkenazi Jewish descent, where the probability of inheriting this mutation is 1 in 10 as compared to 1 in 100 among the general population (National Gaucher Foundation, 2018). Certain genetic diseases can be observed where genetic drift is attributed. This is due to certain genotypes' occurring more frequently within specific groups of people, and the most common reason is referred to as the "founder effect." When a population becomes smaller and isolated over a period of time, genetic variability begins to decline and mutations in the gene pool become more significant as there is a greater chance of passing these mutations to the next generation (National Gaucher Foundation, 2018). Some researchers believe

there can be benefits of the founder effect's occuring within a specific population, such as becoming a carrier to a genetic disease could offer protection against other genetic conditions. For example, being a carrier of sickle cell anemia could not only protect you against malaria but also make it easier to survive if malaria were contracted, which "certainly is an evolutionary advantage" (National Gaucher Foundation, 2018).

- **Natural selection and gene flow**: Genetic variation demonstrates that some traits are more likely to survive and reproduce than others. Charles Darwin eloquently popularized the phrase "survival of the fittest" as a mechanism for natural selection, which is a major evolutionary force driving evolutionary change. These genes are better suited and "survive" environmental change, and these genes are then passed down to the next generation. Natural selection usually predominates in large populations, whereas genetic drift does so in small populations. Gene flow (also referred to as gene migration) most commonly occurs through migration, with the transfer of genetic material from one population to another within the same specifics, and is also mediated by reproduction. Gene flow and natural selection are two central evolutionary forces, sometimes opposing forces since natural selection reduces genetic variation for survival and reproduction whereas gene flow helps distribute genetic variants throughout populations through mechanisms of migration.

### Essential Facts

- Genetic variation within a population enables some to survive better than others in the environment in which they live.
- Genetic drift can cause a population to become genetically distinct from its original population, which could play a role in the evolution of new species.
- Evolutionary forces (mutations, genetic drift, migration, and selection) are mechanisms that facilitate evolutionary change over time.

## DIFFERING POPULATIONS THAT FACILITATE GENETIC DISCOVERY

Genetic variation and diversity have led to there being many populations all around the world. For thousands of years, the genome has evolved and adapted as populations have traveled outside of Africa and been subjected to migration, genetic drift, and natural selection. Africa is considered to be the most genetically diverse continent since this is where *Homo sapiens* are believed to have originated (Yu et al.,

2002). Populations are considered either genetically diverse or isolate, and occur either by choice or by circumstance. ***Isolate*** populations have reduced genetic variation and diversity, leading to increased genetic homogeneity. There are several different isolate types: ethnic, geographic, linguistic, cultural, and religious. In any of these types, increased genetic homogeneity leads to rare variants' becoming more enriched or prevalent, as seen, for example, in the Finnish, Amish, and Greek isolate populations (Hatzikotoulas et al., 2014). Some isolate populations exist where genetic relatedness or sharing of a blood relationship with another person descended from at least one common ancestor (e.g., consanguinity) is common practice, which elevates homogeneity and leads to longer runs of homozygosity within their population as compared to other populations. For example, Middle East populations have shown a higher level of consanguinity; therefore, they share more homogeneity in representing rare variants within their population (Gurdasani et al., 2019; Yang et al., 2014).

Diverse populations have higher levels of genetic variation among individuals, which permits flexibility for survival and adaptability under different environmental circumstances. As populations settled in other parts of the world, various subpopulations were created. ***Admixed*** populations possess ancestry from multiple source groups (e.g., previously diverged or isolated genetic lineages mix) and result from the fusion of populations that have been separated for long periods of time. This admixture leads to the introduction of new genetic lineages into a population. These genomes of individuals from an admixed population have a mosaic of haplotypes from different ancestral origins that can lead to opportunities to assess the association between local ancestry and disease (Gurdasani et al., 2019). These findings can help improve applications for disease mapping and use of personalized medicine across diverse populations. Admixed populations such as African Americans and Hispanic Americans are often medically underserved and have a disproportionately high burden of disease. The use of disease mapping is an important tool in the management of disease and can help raise awareness and make clear to healthcare practitioners the importance of the applicability of genomic medicine within these subpopulations.

## Essential Facts

- Isolate populations have less genetic diversity and more homogeneity. Rare variants become more prevalent among these subpopulations.
- Admixed populations have greater genetic diversity and lead to the creation of new genetic lineages.

## HEALTH EFFECTS DUE TO ENVIRONMENTAL EXPOSURES

Whether a population is considered isolate or genetically diverse, the health effects can be observed at a local, regional, and even global scale. There are health implications to both types of populations as far as the benefits and/or dangers of living either in isolation or in large, diverse communities. For example, regardless of whether it's an isolate or admixed population, living with high levels of air pollution can induce epigenetic alterations (i.e., DNA methylation of specific biomarkers), which can lead to an increase in inflammation, disease development, and exacerbation of risk (i.e., respiratory infections and diseases) (Kim et al., 2018). Isolate populations tend to be more shielded and protected against epidemics and pandemics yet have decreased herd immunity and no antibodies with which to fight against foreign pathogens when introduced for the first time into their population.

## GENETIC-ASSOCIATED DISEASES AMONG HIGH-RISK GROUPS

The World Health Organization (WHO) has stated that genetics plays a substantial role in contributing to the burden of a variety of diseases (WHO Regional Office for South-East Asia, 2010), and further noted that over 20% of the global disease burden and deaths were attributed to modifiable environmental factors (2017). Disease clusters are found all over the world where greater than the expected number of cases occurs within a group of people in a geographic area over a period of time. **Endemic disease clusters** (e.g., always present in a certain population or region) are characteristics of a particular population or region that can be caused by environmental and/or genetic factors, such as a bottleneck or founder effects, decreased gene flow and migration, and inbreeding (e.g., consanguinity), which can lead to inherited recessive diseases that can vary from mild to severe. Therefore, it's important in healthcare to identify global health disparities and address these differences across populations. Healthcare disparities exist due to differences in access or availability to appropriate medical facilities and services, and these disparities vary with different rates of disease occurrence between populations (Agency for Healthcare Research and Quality, n.d.).

One such example are the high rates of *thalassemia and sickle-cell disease*, which are considered the two most common inherited recessive hemoglobin disorders in the world. The highest percentages of cases are most commonly found in the Middle East and North African regions and in individuals of African, Mediterranean, Asian, and Middle Eastern descent. However, due to migration, cases of thalassemia and sickle-cell disease are now found throughout the world (Anwar et al., 2014). Both of these diseases are considered severe because the different mutations found in the *hemoglobin subunit beta (HBB)* gene starves the body of oxygen, leading to shortness of breath, severe tiredness, irregular heartbeats/palpitations, weakness, and a shortage of red blood cells carrying iron throughout the body, which in most cases leads to severe anemia. Without appropriate treatment and disease management, both conditions can be fatal. In the United States, it is estimated that sickle-cell disease affects approximately 100,000 Americans, or approximately 8% of African Americans, occurring in about 1 out of every 365 Black or African American births, and in 1 out of 16,300 Hispanic American births (CDC, 2020). However, thalassemia only affects 1 out of every 100,000 Americans.

In eastern Mediterranean areas, consanguineous marriages continue to be favorably looked upon, with rates considered high among six eastern Mediterranean countries (ranging from 16.5% to 55%) (Hamamy & Alwan, 1994). This practice can lead to genetic diseases' becoming more prevalent. An example includes *familial Mediterranean fever (FMF)*, a rare autoinflammatory syndrome almost always restricted to Turkish, Armenian, Arab, and non–Ashkenazi Jewish heritage, in which one mutant copy has been detected in one of every five people, therefore creating many more carriers among this population. (National Organization for Rare Disorders, n.d.). FMF is caused by mutations in the *MEFV* gene which can lead to deficient levels of the protein pyrin being developed. This hereditary, autosomal recessive disease causes reactive amyloidosis, which can damage the renal and gastrointestinal tracts (Anwar et al., 2014). The goal of treatment for FMF is to control symptoms, because there is no cure for this condition. If caught early enough, a medication called colchicine can be prescribed and has been shown to be effective in preventing the accumulation of amyloid in the kidneys (National Organization for Rare Disorders, n.d.).

*Cystic fibrosis (CF)* is a rare, autosomal recessive genetic disease that mostly affects Caucasians of northern European ancestry. This disease has become such a prevalent inherited genetic disorder among Caucasians living in the United States that it has become standard-of-care practice to screen newborns. Newborn screening is considered a public health service and is required by law prior to a newborn's leaving the hospital. A blood sample is taken from the heel and used to check for a variety of rare genetic, hormone-related, and metabolic conditions, one of which is cystic fibrosis. About 30,000 people in the United States have CF, which equates to about 1 in every 2,500 to 3,500 Caucasian newborns, as compared to 1 in every 17,000 African Americans and 1 in every 100,000 Asian Americans. It's also estimated that 10,500 people in the United Kingdom have the disease, 4,000 Canadians, and 3,300 Australians (National Center for Advancing Translational Sciences [NCATS], n.d.). The chances of being a carrier for CF is 1 in 29 for Caucasian Americans, 1 in 46 for Hispanic Americans, 1 in 65 for African Americans, and 1 in 90 for Asian Americans (NCATS, n.d.). The most commonly affected gene is the *cystic fibrosis transmembrane regulator (CFTR),* which provides instructions to the *CFTR* protein that acts as a channel allowing cells to release chloride and other ions. In individuals with CF, this protein becomes defective and the cells are unable to release chloride, leading to an improper salt balance. This then creates thick, sticky mucus that builds up in the lungs, causing breathing difficulties, inflammation, and bacteria growth, leading to infections. Treatment aims to relieve symptoms through the use of respiratory therapies, medication, and nutritional supplements.

The Indigenous population within the United States is almost exclusively affected by a rare genetic disorder called *Native American myopathy (NAM)*, an inherited recessive disease that encompasses a large and diverse group of diseases defined as a muscle disease due to muscle fibers' not contracting appropriately. Indigenous Americans have one of the highest rates of any form of myopathy among any ethnic group, and data suggests individuals with blood lines to tribes located in the southern half of the United States are more susceptible to carrying NAM than are northern U.S. tribes. Currently, 1 in every 5,000 in the Lumbee Tribe has NAM (Raade & Mandal, 2018). The mutated *STAC3* gene has been associated with congenital myopathy and musculoskeletal involvement of the trunk and extremities, and can lead to feeding difficulties and delayed motor milestones (Webb et al., 1993). NAM is classified as a *STAC3* disorder, and there is currently no treatment, halting, or reversing of the manifestations caused by the mutated *STAC3* gene. However, there is a variety of treatment options to help alleviate neuromuscular symptoms that involve a multidisciplinary team approach.

## Essential Facts

- Endemic disease clusters have a higher prevalence of disease in a population within a geographic area.
- Each population has different health disparities and can be considered high risk for specific genetic-related diseases.

## TARGETED GENETIC EDUCATION

There are well over 6,000 known genetic disorders, with new genomic discoveries constantly being described in our medical literature as our science and technology continue to advance. There is demand for appropriate, needs-based genetic education at all levels, and for more effort being put toward translation and integration into clinical practice and population health. It's becoming increasingly more important for genomic information to be communicated, especially in medically underserved and high-risk populations. Genomic-related health literacy (e.g., knowledge, oral literacy) has been shown to be a critical prerequisite for appropriate care in patients, specifically those with genetic disorders, and in the development of educational strategies that promote communicating genomic information equitably (Kaphingst et al., 2016).

Family history is an important component of understanding the risk of disease, and is a contributing factor to many illnesses and diseases. Patients with inherited diseases are provided genetic education that often entails genetic screening, counseling, treatment-focused genetic testing, and in some cases with family planning that can lead to carrier screening, gene therapy, and other targeted treatments within genetic and disease prevention. Increasing education and awareness of genomic disorders and disease risk will help practitioners and researchers better understand the relationships between genetic traits and diseases across populations. Developing and implementing targeted genetic education will help develop strategies that will promote health and prevent disease, especially among high-risk and underserved populations.

The National Human Genome Research Institute has compiled a list of resources that can be used in a clinical setting by both nongenetics and genetics healthcare professionals with the goal to increasingly use knowledge about genomics to meet the needs of their patients (NHGRI, 2021). These resources include professional genomic competencies required for specific disciplines and teaching resources for the virtual or in-person classroom. Healthcare providers, nurses, educators, and society representatives can further professional genomics education through a wide variety of modalities and frameworks, including (not limited to) in-person trainings, calls/webinars, and peer-reviewed curricula. Genetic and genomic case studies and videos are available to students and practicing healthcare professionals to help them learn basic genetic and genomic concepts. Published guidelines and core competencies are available for practicing healthcare professionals across a wide spectrum of medical disciplines that consist of a basic set of genomic skills to support gathering a family history, genomic testing, treatment based on genomic results, somatic genomics, and microbial genomic information. Lastly, opportunities exist for healthcare practitioners to collaborate across disciplines with the understanding that genomics health literacy, targeted education, and communication are vital for improving the overall health and well-being of patients living with genomic disorders across populations.

## CONCLUSION

Population-based genetics is the study of genetic variation within and among populations, and how evolutionary forces can modify these genes over a period of time, which can lead to evolutionary changes within a population, specifically genetic-associated diseases among high-risk groups. Major scientific and medical achievements and breakthroughs have led to further understanding of how genes influence an individual's disease etiology, risk, and management. Our genomes contain evolutionary histories that can provide either an evolutionary advantage or disadvantage. Genomic variation within species can be analyzed using various genomic analysis tools to help explain these relationships. The Human Genome Project along with many other technological advancements has provided us with an immeasurable opportunity to enhance our understanding of our genome and its implications for medicine. Population-based genetics has changed the landscape of how we can retrieve and utilize genetic information to inform diagnostic and therapeutic modalities. This is crucial in forecasting future disease risk and how this can lead to improved patient care with disease monitoring, treatment decisions, and disease prevention.

## REFERENCES

Agency for Healthcare Research and Quality. (n.d.). *Disparities*. https://www.ahrq.gov/topics/disparities.html

Anwar, W. A., Khyatti, M., & Hemminki, K. (2014). Consanguinity and genetic diseases in North Africa and immigrants to Europe. *European Journal of Public Health*, *24*(suppl 1), 57–63. https://doi.org/10.1093/eurpub/cku104

Benton, M. L., Abraham, A., LaBella, A. L., Abbot, P., Rokas, A., & Capra, J. A. (2021). The influence of evolutionary history on human health and disease. *Nature Reviews Genetics*, *22*(5), 269–283. https://doi.org/10.1038/s41576-020-00305-9

Cargill, M., Altshuler, D., Ireland, J., Sklar, P., Ardlie, K., Patil, N., Lane, C. R., Lim, E. P., Kalyanaraman, N., Nemesh, J., Ziaugra, L., Friedland, L., Rolfe, A., Warrington, J., Lipshutz, R., Daley, G. Q., & Lander, E. S. (1999). Characterization of single-nucleotide polymorphisms in coding regions of human genes. *Nature Genetics, 22*(3), 231–238. https://doi.org/10.1038/10290

Centers for Disease Control and Prevention. (2017). *Population research.* https://www.cdc.gov/genomics/population/index.htm

Centers for Disease Control and Prevention. (2020). *Data & statistics on sickle cell disease.* https://www.cdc.gov/ncbddd/sicklecell/data.html

Coppola, L., Cianflone, A., Grimaldi, A. M., Incoronato, M., Bevilacqua, P., Messina, F., Baselice, S., Soricelli, A., Mirabelli, P., & Salvatore, M. (2019). Biobanking in health care: Evolution and future directions. *Journal of Translational Medicine, 17*(1), 172. https://doi.org/10.1186/s12967-019-1922-3

Evans, O., & Manchanda, R. (2020). Population-based genetic testing for precision prevention. *Cancer Prevention Research, 13*(8), 643–648. https://doi.org/10.1158/1940-6207.CAPR-20-0002

Gurdasani, D., Barroso, I., Zeggini, E., & Sandhu, M. S. (2019). Genomics of disease risk in globally diverse populations. *Nature Reviews Genetics, 20*(9), 520–535. https://doi.org/10.1038/s41576-019-0144-0

Hamamy, H., & Alwan, A. (1994). Hereditary disorders in the Eastern Mediterranean region. *Bulletin of the World Health Organization, 72*(1), 145–154.

Hatzikotoulas, K., Gilly, A., & Zeggini, E. (2014). Using population isolates in genetic association studies. *Briefings in Functional Genomics, 13*(5), 371–377. https://doi.org/10.1093/bfgp/elu022

Kaphingst, K. A., Blanchard, M., Milam, L., Pokharel, M., Elrick, A., & Goodman, M. S. (2016). Relationships between health literacy and genomics-related knowledge, self-efficacy, perceived importance, and communication in a medically underserved population. *Journal of Health Communication, 21*(Suppl 1), 58–68. https://doi.org/10.1080/10810730.2016.1144661

Kim, D., Chen, Z., Zhou, L.-F., & Huang, S.-X. (2018). Air pollutants and early origins of respiratory diseases. *Chronic Diseases and Translational Medicine, 4*(2), 75–94. https://doi.org/10.1016/j.cdtm.2018.03.003

Lu, Y.-F., Goldstein, D. B., Angrist, M., & Cavalleri, G. (2014). Personalized medicine and human genetic diversity. *Cold Spring Harbor Perspectives in Medicine, 4*(9), a008581. https://doi.org/10.1101/cshperspect.a008581

National Center for Advancing Translational Sciences. (n.d.). *Cystic fibrosis.* https://rarediseases.info.nih.gov/diseases/6233/cystic-fibrosis

National Gaucher Foundation. (2018). *The founder effect's influence on Jewish genetic diseases.* https://www.gaucherdisease.org/blog/founder-effects-influence-jewish-genetic-diseases/

National Human Genome Research Institute. (n.d.). *Genetic variation.* https://www.genome.gov/genetics-glossary/Genetic-Variation

National Human Genome Research Institute. (2020). *Genome-wide association studies fact sheet.* https://www.genome.gov/about-genomics/fact-sheets/Genome-Wide-Association-Studies-Fact-Sheet

National Human Genome Research Institute. (2021). *Healthcare provider genomics education resources.* https://www.genome.gov/For-Health-Professionals/Provider-Genomics-Education-Resources

National Organization for Rare Disorders. (n.d.). *Familial Mediterranean fever.* https://rarediseases.org/rare-diseases/familial-mediterranean-fever/

Raade, E. J., & Mandal, K. P. (2018). Major health issues of American Indians. *Journal of Applied Biotechnology & Bioengineering, 5*(3), 188–191. https://doi.org/10.15406/jabb.2018.05.00136

Saint Pierre, A., & Genin, E. (2014). How important are rare variants in common disease? *Briefings in Functional Genomics, 13*(5), 353–361. https://doi.org/10.1093/bfgp/elu025

The 1000 Genomes Project. (2011). Variation in genome-wide mutation rates within and between human families. *Nature Genetics, 43*(7), 712–714. https://doi.org/10.1038/ng.862

Webb, B. D., Manoli, I., & Jabs, E. W. (1993). STAC3 disorder. In M. P. Adam, H. H. Ardinger, R. A. Pagon, S. E. Wallace, L. J. Bean, G. Mirzaa, & A. Amemiya (Eds.), *GeneReviews®. University of Washington, Seattle. http://www.ncbi.nlm.nih.gov/books/NBK542808/*

World Health Organization Regional Office for South-East Asia. (2010). *Regional health forum, Vol. 14, No. 1.* Author. https://apps.who.int/iris/handle/10665/205781

Yang, X., Al-Bustan, S., Feng, Q., Guo, W., Ma, Z., Marafie, M., Jacob, S., Al-Mulla, F., & Xu, S. (2014). The influence of admixture and consanguinity on population genetic diversity in Middle East. *Journal of Human Genetics, 59*(11), 615–622. https://doi.org/10.1038/jhg.2014.81

Yu, N., Chen, F.-C., Ota, S., Jorde, L. B., Pamilo, P., Patthy, L., Ramsay, M., Jenkins, T., Shyue, S.-K., & Li, W.-H. (2002). Larger genetic differences within Africans than between Africans and Eurasians. *Genetics, 161*(1), 269–274.

# 13

# Pharmacogenomics

Dennis Cheek

*For many years the utilization of drugs in the treatment of disease was based upon trial and error with significant adverse drug reaction. Since the completion of the Human Genome Project in 2003 and the more recent Personal Medicine Initiative from the White House in 2015, the drug regime has undergone a significant revision. The identification of numerous genetic targets along with the growing availability of genetic testing has led to the development of pharmacogenomics. Drugs can now be targeted to patients' genetic makeup, thus improving the drug's efficacy along with reducing adverse drug reactions.*

**In this chapter, you will learn:**

1. The difference is between pharmacogenetics and pharmacogenomics
2. The role of pharmacogenomics and the CYP450 metabolizing system
3. The role of the nurse in pharmacogenomics and the patient medication regime

The International Human Genome Sequencing Consortium announced on April 14, 2003, the successful completion of the Human Genome Project (International Consortium Completes Human Genome Project, 2003). In January 2015, the White House announced the Precision Medicine Initiative, with a focus on the individual genetic/genomic makeup, environment, and lifestyles (Denny & Collins, 2021; Precision Medicine Initiative, 2015). The established approach with drug therapy has been based upon the "average person," and trial and error is now being challenged and giving way to an innovative approach that takes into account the person's genetics or pharmacogenomics.

## PHARMACOGENOMICS

*Pharmacogenetics* and *pharmacogenomics* are terms often used when describing the variation of a drug response based on a patient's DNA. The term *pharmacogenetics* describes a study for a specific gene or set of genes involved in a drug response (McInnes & Altman, 2021). With advancing technology used in detecting genetic markers, pharmacogenomics has become an emerging field of genomic medicine in which healthcare professionals can use the patient's whole genome to identify the appropriate drug therapy. Because a single gene rarely causes most drug responses, a comprehensive approach of scanning the entire genome in combination with looking at environmental influences is a better method to personalize treatment.

With the completion of the human genome sequencing project in 2003, researchers and clinicians now understand that more than 99.9% of all genetic material is identical. Differences among individuals are caused by less than 0.1% of a person's DNA (Zerbino et al., 2020). The basic components of the DNA sequence are a phosphate group, sugars, and four nucleotides—adenine, cytosine, guanine, and thymine (also referred to as the letters A, C, G, and T). Phosphate groups and sugars make up the backbone of the DNA. The nucleotides are bound to these sugars through bonds to form a single strand. For DNA to form a double-strand helix, two opposite strands have to bind together through the attachment of nucleotides, which is referred to as base pairing. This base pairing occurs with the joining of adenine and thymine, as well as the binding of cytosine and guanine (Watson & Crick, 1974).

The sequences of DNA are broken into genes, which hold the information for the protein sequences. The structure of a gene sequence consists of exons, introns, and promoter regions. The exons, or coding regions, contain the genetic information needed for the protein sequence. The introns are the spaces found between the exons of a gene. The promoter region plays an important role in initiating the process for sending the message of protein translation (Zerbino et al., 2020). The process of translating the DNA into a protein starts with the unwinding of the DNA helix. The DNA is then separated into single strands, and an enzyme, called an RNA polymerase, attaches to the promoter region. The nucleotides are transcribed into messenger RNA (mRNA), and thymine in the mRNA is replaced by uracil (U). Once the message is complete, the mRNA is released from the DNA as a single-stranded sequence, with the exon and intron segments. The intron segments are then removed through a splicing process. Once the splicing process is complete, the mRNA containing only the exon sequence is ready for translation (Zerbino et al., 2020).

The strand of mRNA is read in triplets (called codons); for example, "AUCCGTATA" is read as "AUC CGT ATA," translated by a ribosome complex into strings of amino acids, which are cut by enzymes once the protein sequence is complete. The "codon spelling" of amino acids can have one or several triplet spellings.

Polymorphisms, or variants, are the genetic changes that make the population diverse and also cause every individual to have a unique genomic sequence. Several different types of polymorphisms exist, such as single-nucleotide polymorphisms (SNPs, pronounced "snips") or single-nucleotide variants (SNV), copy number variants, and repeated sequences (Kitts et al., 2013; Ormond et al., 2021). A SNP/SNV is a single nucleotide change that occurs in a particular position of the DNA sequence. This could be the difference of adenine replaced by thymine, or cytosine replaced by guanine, on the genomic sequence. These simple changes could have great or limited effect based on where the nucleotide substitution occurs in the triplet codon or the type of nucleotide change. All referenced SNPs are cataloged by the Short Genetic Variations database, known as dbSNP (Kitts et al., 2013). The SNPs in this database are given a reference ID number, or rs number. For example, the CYP450s are a group of heme-conforming enzymes responsible for phase I metabolic reactions. The *CYP2D6* gene has a SNP in the coding region referenced as rs28371703, which is a missense variant, which is a point mutation in which a single-nucleotide change results in a codon that codes for a different amino acid.

**Essential Facts**

Single-nucleotide polymorphism (SNP) or single-nucleotide variants (SNV) are a single-nucleotide change that occurs in a particular position of the DNA sequence.

## CYTOCHROME P-450 SYSTEM

The successful sequencing of the human genome in 2003 has further elucidated the two processes common to pharmacology. Pharmacokinetics (PK) focuses on the movement of drugs in the body from entrance to exit by studying the absorption, distribution, metabolism, and excretion of the drug. Absorption describes how much drug is available in the vascular system for distribution and use by the cells. Enzymes participate in the metabolic transformation of the drug structure by changing it into an active or inactive form. The drug and its metabolites are removed from the body via excretion. Thus, PK determines the concentration of drug available for attachment to the targeted proteins and the uptake of the drug by the cells. Any genetic variation to the PK process can affect how an individual will respond to medication; this could lead to a decrease in efficacy or an increase in side effects (Klomp et al., 2020; Song et al., 2021). Pharmacodynamics (PD) is the study of what a drug does to the body through the binding of direct and indirect targets. These targets include receptors, enzymes, signal proteins, and other interactions. Physiologic changes influenced by disorders, aging, and other drugs can affect the PD (Klomp et al., 2020).

Drug metabolism converts foreign substances, known as xenobiotics, into active drug or water-soluble metabolites that are more easily excreted (Klomp et al., 2020). Typically, the pathways of metabolism are classified as either phase I or phase II. Phase I reactions consist of oxidation, reduction, and hydrolysis of the drug via the CYP450 enzymes. In most cases, these reactions lead to the active metabolism of drugs (Bakar, 2021). Phase II reactions are typically responsible for detoxification (or inactivation) of drugs and other ingested molecules.

The cytochrome P 450s (CYP 450s) are a group of heme-conforming enzymes responsible for phase I metabolic reactions. Fifty-seven of the CYP genes are designated as individual families based on their similarity in the positions of amino acids (International Consortium Completes Human Genome Project, 2003). The CYP label indicates a human cytochrome. This designation is followed by the family number (CYP1, CYP2), a capital letter for the subfamily (CYP2A), and a second number to identify the gene coding the enzyme (*CYP2A3*). The most common type is designated as *1 (e.g., *CYP2A3*1*). Any other variation is assigned *2, *3, and so on, depending on the number of SNPs that have been identified in the gene. If an unexpected drug response is associated with a SNP variation, it would be noted as *CYP2A3*2*, or for a different drug response with another SNP variation, the notation would be *CYP2A3*3*. For example, a recent research study identified that individuals with a variation in *CYP2D6*4* had low or no enzyme activity. An example of the *CYP2D6*4* variation is women treated with tamoxifen were found to be at a higher risk for a relapse (Province et al., 2014).

The CYP enzymes have the ability to activate or inactivate drugs. A CYP enzyme with the ability to "inhibit" will prevent or decrease the activity of the drug. This means if the drug is not degraded or inactivated, more drug is available, which may cause increased toxicities for the patient. Other CYP enzymes "induce," or increase, the enzyme activity. If more of the drug is deactivated, then less of the drug is available for therapeutic effect.

**Essential Facts**

2D6 *1/*1 or *2/*2 – Wildtype (WT)-Normal metabolizer (NM)
2D6 *3/*4/*5/*6 – Poor metabolizer (PM)
2D6 *7/*10/*41 – Intermediate metabolizer (IM)

## PHARMACOGENOMICS AND ONCOLOGY

To better understand the role of pharmacogenomics in oncology nursing, it is important to review key terminology and concepts (Cheek & Howington, 2018). Genetic variation in cancer also can change the PD through receptor binding (such as *BCR-ABL* translocation), increased levels of binding proteins (such as HER2/neu overexpression), and decreased receptor sensitivity (Schmidt et al., 2016). If it is a chemotherapy agent, the patient may receive a lesser amount of the drug than needed to combat the cancer (Schmidt et al., 2016). The SNPs in genes can code for other metabolizing drug enzymes besides the CYP enzymes. Two non-CYP drug-metabolizing proteins include a phase I metabolizer, dihydropyrimidine dehydrogenase (DPD), and a phase II metabolizer, thiopurine methyl-transferase (TPMT). Like the CYP enzymes, these can affect the toxicities and efficacy of anticancer drugs and their side effects (Relling et al., 2019; Root et al., 2020; Schmidt et al., 2016).

A commonly used chemotherapy agent, 5-fluorouracil (5-FU), is inactivated to a metabolite by the DPD enzyme coded from *DYPD*. The activity of this gene product (enzyme) has been associated with up to 20-fold differences in drug metabolism among humans. The *DYPD*2A* is found over the exon–intron junction (referred to as a *splice site modification*) and is associated with low (heterozygous—one allele has *2A) or no (homozygous—both alleles have *2A) enzyme activity. Patients with low or no enzyme activity who are treated with 5-FU will accumulate active metabolites, causing a significantly greater risk of hematopoietic, neurologic, and gastrointestinal toxicities, which can be fatal. Genetic testing for the gene causing the enzyme deficiency prior to receiving 5-FU treatment is commercially available (Schmidt et al., 2016).

As a phase II metabolizing drug, 6-mercaptopurine (6-MP) is catalyzed by TPMT to form inactive metabolites so that antimetabolites do not incorporate into the DNA or RNA of healthy cells. Three main variants (*3A, *3B, and *3C) are associated with low levels of TPMT enzymatic activity. If a patient possesses one of these variants (heterozygous), less drug degradation and increased toxicities will occur and the patient would need some reduction in dosage. If the patient has two of the same variants (homozygosity), he or she may require significant dose reductions or alternative treatment options (Relling et al., 2019; Schmidt et al., 2016). In the United States, 10% of Caucasians and African Americans have intermediate (heterozygous) TPMT activity. One in 300 individuals has low or undetectable (homozygous) TPMT activity (Schmidt et al., 2016). Applying this information to a patient situation, a young child being treated for acute lymphoblastic leukemia could receive 6-MP. If this child has low TPMT enzyme activity, life-threatening neutropenia and thrombocytopenia could occur (Relling et al., 2019; Schmidt et al., 2016). Prospective genetic testing is available to identify members of this at-risk population. Children who experience myelosuppression after their initial dose of 6-MP should be considered for genetic testing (Relling et al., 2019; Schmidt et al., 2016).

Another phase II metabolizer, UDP-glycosyltransferase 1A1 (UGT1A1), is associated with devastating toxicities for patients who are either homozygous or heterozygous for the *UGT1A1*28* allele. This variant is a sequence of seven TA nucleotide repeats in the promoter region of the *UGT1A1* gene versus the six repeats in the wild-type sequence. Individuals with the variant can have 1,000-fold greater inhibition of topoisomerase, causing diarrhea and leukopenia when dosed with irinotecan. In addition, unconjugated serum bilirubin levels are increased. Genetic testing is available, but it has not been confirmed that dose reduction based on test results will not affect the efficacy of treatment (Relling et al., 2019; Schmidt et al., 2016).

## PHARMACOGENOMICS AND MENTAL HEALTH

The World Health Organization (WHO) estimates that about 25% of the population around the world will suffer from at least one mental disorder at some time in their lives (Wainberg et al., 2017). Depression and anxiety are among the most common disorders, and these can affect people regardless of age, gender, ethnicity, or background. We do not fully understand what causes most cases of mental health problems, but it is known that both genetic and environmental factors can contribute to an individual's predisposition to a particular disorder (Wainberg et al., 2017). Knowledge of human genetics fosters an understanding of pharmacogenomics. Genes encode for the production of metabolism proteins. These metabolic proteins have a dramatic effect on PK, or what the body does to the drug. These metabolism proteins housed within the liver are known as the cytochrome P450 system (CYP450) (Song et al., 2021). Individual differences in the CYP450 genes play a role in the extent of drug metabolism. Classification of individuals may be based upon their genotype as either poor metabolizers, intermediate metabolizers, normal metabolizers, or ultra-rapid metabolizers. In general, the metabolization of psychotropic drugs is through CYP450 systems, and therefore an understanding of the differences between these classifications of metabolizers is critical to understanding why pharmacogenomics can be helpful for purposes of prescribing (Cheek & Howington, 2018; Klomp et al., 2020; Roden et al., 2019).

The differences between these categories are attributable to the influence of alleles, or alternative forms of a gene that result from mutation. If an individual carries a genetic variation, it may result in either increased or decreased clearance of a drug from the body (Cheek & Howington, 2018; Klomp et al., 2020; Roden et al., 2019). To underscore the importance of this knowledge, the amount of drug in the body can lead to more pronounced adverse drug reactions or, alternatively, a lack of therapeutic effect. The ability to genetically test for the presence of alleles is achieved through exploration of an individual's CYP450 metabolic profile (Cheek & Howington, 2018; Klomp et al., 2020; Roden et al., 2019).

The differences between these categories can be conceptualized as a continuum of drug metabolism, where the poles represent slow and rapid (Cheek & Howington, 2018; Klomp et al., 2020; Roden et al., 2019). Poor metabolizers are slow washout, meaning that more drug may accrue in the system, leading to a greater potential for adverse reactions. Intermediate metabolizers are slower than normal, and because of this may require a decreased dose of a drug. Extensive/normal metabolizers break down drugs at a normal rate, and therefore may take the standard amount of medication. Ultra-rapid metabolizers lie at the fast end of the spectrum and may need a higher than normal dosage due to increased clearance of the drug from the system.

The CYP450 system has more than 57 variants of metabolic enzymes (Klomp et al., 2020; Song et al., 2021; Wainberg et al., 2017). Of these, two (CYP2D6 and CYP2C19) are crucial for the processing of psychotropic drugs such as antidepressants and antipsychotics (PharmGKB.org, 2021). These two classes of pharmacotherapies are notorious for adverse drug reactions. Notably, antipsychotics can cause a wide array of side effects, including tardive dyskinesia, akathisia, weight gain, and decreased insulin sensitivity, among others (Klomp et al., 2020; Song et al., 2021; Wainberg et al., 2017). Most genetic variations in *CYP2D6* and *CYP2C19* may lead to a reduction in enzyme activity, but a few can cause increased enzyme activity. Another important reason for pharmacogenomic testing is that many individuals are prescribed antidepressants for reasons other than depression, and therefore the scope of the need for genetic testing is widened (Roden et al., 2019).

## PHARMACOGENOMICS AND NURSING IMPLICATIONS

As of August 20, 2021, the FDA lists over 483 entries for numerous drugs for which there are molecular biomarkers that may aid in achieving better therapeutic outcomes for patients carrying these genetic markers (FDA, 2021). The therapeutic area for which there are the most pharmacogenetic indications (30%) is oncology, largely due to the narrow therapeutic indices typical of most oncology drugs. To facilitate the clinical application of pharmacogenomic data, the Clinical Pharmacogenetics Implementation Consortium (CPIC) was formed in 2009. The CPIC regularly publishes and updates peer-reviewed gene/drug clinical guidelines in the journal *Clinical Pharmacology and Therapeutics* (CPIC, 2021). Similarly, the Royal Dutch Pharmacist's Association (KNMP) has developed pharmacogenetics-based therapeutic recommendations based upon extensive reviews of the literature (Abdullah-Koolmees et al., 2021).

Perhaps the best source for timely information concerning genetic polymorphisms and drug response is the databases accessible via the Internet. Two databases with the most comprehensive, up-to-date, and trustworthy pharmacogenomic/pharmacogenetic data are the National Center for Biotechnology Information (NCBI at www.ncbi.nlm.nih.gov) and the Pharmacogenomics and Pharmacogenetics Knowledge Base (PharmGKB at www.PharmGKB.org). Both databases have helpful online tutorials and glossaries for navigating through the immense data, and both are free to the public. The importance of these databases cannot be overemphasized. Given the speed at which the field of pharmacogenomics is growing and the amount of data that are being generated, these databases are indispensable resources for up-to-date pharmacogenomic information.

The NCBI at the National Institutes of Health was created in 1988 to be the repository for all molecular and genetic data. It is the most comprehensive starting point for any search of molecular biology information and human health (NCBI, 2021). While NCBI has a great many individual databases, the one database that may be of most interest to health professionals is the Online Mendelian Inheritance in Man (OMIM) database. OMIM is the repository for all data concerning human genes and genetic diseases. As of 2021 the database has records for over 24,597 human genes. OMIM has textual information with links to MEDLINE and all the many additional related databases and resources at NCBI, including sequence data, genetic maps, and SNP data. OMIM is searchable by disease name, gene name, or drug. OMIM is designed for use primarily by healthcare professionals, though some knowledge of genetic terminology and concepts is essential.

The Pharmacogenomics and Pharmacogenetics Knowledge Base is an integrated database providing clinical, pharmacokinetic, pharmacodynamic, genotypic, and molecular function data for human genetic polymorphisms and drugs (Whirl-Carrillo et al., 2021). Like NCBI, PharmGKB is free and open to the public. PharmGKB is the best source for up-to-date information concerning individual genes and drug response. This database has been developed and maintained by Stanford University to aid researchers in assessing the nature of genetic variation among individuals and how this variation contributes to differences in patient response to drugs. The PharmGKB has been established to allow researchers and health professionals to easily access current data on drugs and genetic variability at a number of levels. Like the information at NCBI, these data represent the most current information available, but in order to make the most of the information some understanding of genetic principles is necessary.

## CONCLUSION

Genetics is an increasingly complex field of medicine. Nurses need to understand basic pharmacogenomics in order to educate patients about the importance of family history as relates to typical and unexpected drug responses, the rationale for differences in drugs and drug doses between patients with the same cancer diagnosis, and the need to report unexpected side effects.

The implications of pharmacogenomics on nursing practice are significant. No longer will drugs be prescribed for the general public on a trial-and-error basis, but rather a specific drug will be utilized for a specific patient genotype, resulting in personalized medicine.

Not only are nurses responsible for providing high-quality care to their patient, but they are also responsible for the ongoing assessment of medication therapy. They are responsible for the administration of the various drugs ordered for the patient, always monitoring the efficacy of the drug as well as any potential adverse drug reactions. With the completion of the Human Genome Project there has been a significant growth of genetic-genomic knowledge, which is being translated into drug therapy (PharmGKB.org). The nurse of the future will need to review not only drug information sheets, but also lab data, including genetic-genomic profiles of their patient, prior to the administration of prescribed medication. The nurse is in the ideal position to implement the pharmacogenomics principles, reduce adverse drug reactions, facilitate correct drug dosing, and increase the drug efficacy of their patients.

## END-OF-CHAPTER QUESTIONS

1. Compare pharmacogenetics and pharmacogenomics.
2. Describe the cytochrome p 450 system (CYP450).
3. Discuss the common variant being sought when a phamacogenomic testing is ordered.

## REFERENCES

Abdullah-Koolmees, H., van Keulen, A. M., Nijenhuis, M., & Deneer, V. (2021). Pharmacogenetics guidelines: Overview and comparison of the DPWG, CPIC, CPNDS, and RNPGx guidelines. *Frontiers in Pharmacology, 11*, 595219. https://doi.org/10.3389/fphar.2020.595219

Bakar, N. S. (2021). Pharmacogenetics of common SNP affecting drug metabolizing enzymes: Comparison of allele frequencies between European and Malaysian/Singaporean. *Drug Metabolism and Personalized Therapy*, Advance online publication. https://doi.org/10.1515/dmdi-2020-0153

Cheek, D., & Howington, L. (2018). Pharmacogenomics in critical care. *AACN Advanced Critical Care, 29*(1), 36–42. https://doi.org/10.4037/aacnacc2018398

Clinical Pharmacogenetics Implementation Consortium. (2021). *CPIC: Clinical Pharmacogenetics Implementation Consortium*. http://www.pharmgkb.org/page/cpic

Denny, J. C., & Collins, F. S. (2021). Precision medicine in 2030—Seven ways to transform healthcare. *Cell, 184*(6), 1415–1419. https://doi.org/10.1016/j.cell.2021.01.015

FDA. (2021). *Table of pharmacogenomic biomarkers in drug labeling.* https://www.fda.gov/drugs/science-and-research-drugs/table-pharmacogenomic-biomarkers-drug-labeling

International Consortium Completes Human Genome Project. (2003). https://www.genome.gov/11006929/2003-release-international-consortium-completes-HGP

Kitts, A., Phan, L., Ward, M., & Holmes, J. B. (2013). The database of Short Genetic Variation (dbSNP). In: *The NCBI handbook [Internet]* (2nd ed.). National Center for Biotechnology Information (US). https://www.ncbi.nlm.nih.gov/books/NBK174586/

Klomp, S. D., Manson, M. L., Guchelaar, H. J., & Swen, J. J. (2020). Phenoconversion of cytochrome P450 metabolism: A systematic review. *Journal of Clinical Medicine, 9*(9), 2890. https://doi.org/10.3390/jcm9092890

McInnes, G., & Altman, R. (2021). Drug response pharmacogenetics for 200,000 UK biobank participants. *Pacific Symposium on Biocomputing, 26*, 184–195.

National Center for Biotechnology Information, U.S. National Library of Medicine. (2021). *Database of single nucleotide polymorphism (dbSNP).* https://www.ncbi.nlm.nih.gov/snp/

Ormond, C., Ryan, N. M., Corvin, A., & Heron, E. A. (2021). Converting single nucleotide variants between genome builds: From cautionary tale to solution. *Briefings in Bioinformatics*, bbab069. https://doi.org/10.1093/bib/bbab069

PharmGKB.org. (2021). *Overview of PharmGKB.* https://www.pharmgkb.org/

Precision Medicine Initiative. (2015). https://obamawhitehouse.archives.gov/precision-medicine

Province, M. A., Goetz, M. P., Brauch, H., Flockhart, D. A., Hebert, J. M., Whaley, R., Suman, V. J., Schroth, W., Winter, S., Zembutsu, H., Mushiroda, T., Newman, W. G., Lee, M. T., Ambrosone, C. B., Beckmann, M. W., Choi, J. Y., Dieudonné, A. S., Fasching, P. A., Ferraldeschi, R., … International Tamoxifen Pharmacogenomics Consortium. (2014). CYP2D6 genotype and adjuvant tamoxifen: Meta-analysis of heterogeneous study populations. *Clinical Pharmacology and Therapeutics, 95*(2), 216–227. https://doi.org/10.1038/clpt.2013.186

Relling, M. V., Schwab, M., Whirl-Carrillo, M., Suarez-Kurtz, G., Pui, C. H., Stein, C. M., Moyer, A. M., Evans, W. E., Klein, T. E., Antillon-Klussmann, F. G., Caudle, K. E., Kato, M., Yeoh, A., Schmiegelow, K., & Yang, J. J. (2019). Clinical Pharmacogenetics Implementation Consortium guideline for thiopurine dosing based on TPMT and NUDT15 genotypes: 2018 update. *Clinical Pharmacology and Therapeutics, 105*(5), 1095–1105. https://doi.org/10.1002/cpt.1304

Roden, D. M., McLeod, H. L., Relling, M. V., Williams, M. S., Mensah, G. A., Peterson, J. F., & Van Driest, S. L. (2019). Pharmacogenomics. *Lancet, 394*(10197), 521–532. https://doi.org/10.1016/S0140-6736(19)31276-0

Root, A., Johnson, R., McGee, A., Lee, H. J., Yang, S., & Voora, D. (2020). Understanding the state of pharmacogenomic testing for thiopurine methyltransferase within a large health system. *Pharmacogenomics, 21*(6), 411–418. https://doi.org/10.2217/pgs-2019-0148

Schmidt, K. T., Chau, C. H., Price, D. K., & Figg, W. D. (2016). Precision oncology medicine: The clinical relevance of patient-specific biomarkers used to optimize cancer treatment. *Journal of Clinical Pharmacology, 56*(12), 1484–1499. https://doi.org/10.1002/jcph.765

Song, Y., Li, C., Liu, G., Liu, R., Chen, Y., Li, W., Cao, Z., Zhao, B., Lu, C., & Liu, Y. (2021). Drug-metabolizing cytochrome P450 enzymes have multifarious influences on treatment outcomes. *Clinical Pharmacokinetics*, Advance Online Publication. https://doi.org/10.1007/s40262-021-01001-5

Wainberg, M. L., Scorza, P., Shultz, J. M., Helpman, L., Mootz, J. J., Johnson, K. A., Neria, Y., Bradford, J. M. E., Oquendo, M. A., & Arbuckle, M. R. (2017). Challenges and opportunities in global mental health: A research-to-practice perspective. *Current Psychiatry Reports, 19*, 28. https://doi.org/10.1007/s11920-017-0780-z

Watson, J. D., & Crick, F. H. (1974). Molecular structure of nucleic acids: A structure for deoxyribose nucleic acid. Published in *Nature*, 4356 (April 25, 1953). *Nature, 248*(5451), 765. https://doi.org/10.1038/248765a0

Whirl-Carrillo, M., Huddart, R., Gong, L., Sangkuhl, K., Thorn, C. F., Whaley, R., & Klein, T. E. (2021). An evidence-based framework for evaluating pharmacogenomics knowledge for personalized medicine. *Clinical Pharmacology & Therapeutics*. Online ahead of print.

Zerbino, D. R., Frankish, A., & Flicek, P. (2020). Progress, challenges, and surprises in annotating the human genome. *Annual Review of Genomics and Human Genetics, 21*, 55–79. https://doi.org/10.1146/annurev-genom-121119-083418

# 14

# Genetic Technology

Alexandra Noel Grace

*Technology refers to the application of human knowledge to means that result in an enhanced, simplified, or accelerated outcome to the questions and functions of life. Genetic technology is the summation of the genetic tools that serve this purpose. The introductory notion of a gene has long evolved from the 19th-century vision of germplasm to now extraordinarily sophisticated ideas of the genomic structure and tools that can manipulate the genetic code. The field of genetic technology is now shifting its focus to skillfully influencing the fundamental building blocks of life and personalized genomic medicine. All healthcare practitioners need awareness of current genetic technology and what it can offer their patients.*

**In this chapter, you will learn about:**

1. Cloning
2. Stem cell research
3. Genetic modifications in science and medicine
4. Gene editing and CRISPR

To unify the most basic concepts of genetic technology in medicine, it is important to recognize that all living things from microorganisms, plants, insects, and animals, to humans can be individually identified by the makeup that is their DNA. Every cell in multicellular organisms, with the exception of mature red blood cells, contains a copy of its entire genome. The human genome comprises two coiled strands of DNA that are connected by corresponding bonded molecules called nucleotides. Researchers have identified thousands of genes across a multitude of species, and it is estimated that the human genome contains anywhere from 20,000 to 25,000 genes, which, have been found to make up less than 3% of the genome. Each gene can generate RNA, that by way of translation to form a protein, can result in one or more assigned functions. Genes can be turned on or off to express certain functions in cells of the body by epigenetic mechanisms (such as methylation or chromatin remodeling) and environmental factors such as stress, diet, and teratogens. The summation of DNA and cellular expression within a cell is referred to as the epigenome (Simmet et al., 2021). Early research in cloning living organisms gave way to the current knowledge of the epigenome and the fact the DNA is the blueprint of living things.

Scientists have long been intrigued by clones. Simply defined, a clone is one or more offspring that are exact copies of one another. Cloning is a naturally occurring process in a number of lifeforms such as bacteria which reproduce asexually. Similarly, plant propagation is a form of cloning. Given the limitations in scientific knowledge on the molecular mechanisms of biology and reproduction, how identical twins were formed in humans and other organisms remained an unexplained mystery as scientists studied heritability and traits.

The initial notion of the nucleus as reproductive governor was first sensationalized by Hans Spemann, who suggested in 1938 that DNA could be extracted and implanted into enucleated eggs. As there was no actualized basis for this, a consensus on the molecular components of reproduction, inheritance, and chromosomes would not converge until decades later (Gouveia et al., 2020).

The first cloning attempts were achieved in amphibians because, unlike most other species, embryonic frog cells are visible to the naked eye and can be physically manipulated with a micropipette. The first successful efforts to clone an organism were attempted by transferring blastomere nuclei into enucleated eggs in 1952. A decade later, a new process called nuclear transplantation came to be published in 1962. Nuclear transplantation is a method by which a single cell is separated or removed from either an embryo or mature organism and fused into a donor oocyte to create an individual mirrored organism, or twin. A small hole is made prior to the transfer in the donor oocyte to remove its DNA spindle. Experiments conducted by biologist John Gurdon in frogs and tadpoles began to offer insight on the cellular stages of development and the process by which somatic cells are differentiated in a mature organism (Gouveia et al., 2020).

## Essential Facts

One scientific outcome of the first cloning techniques was the acceptance that all living things are formed from a single cell. The first conducting cell in the development of humans and other multicellular organisms is called a zygote. Once created, the zygote will divide to form two blastomere cells, which through the process of complex organization and exponentiation form a subdivided differentiated globe of cells called a blastocyst. In humans and animals, the blastocyst contains three compartments: the embryoblast, the trophoblast, and a blastocystic cavity. Organs will then form the specialized layers of cells from the embryoblast, called the ectoderm, mesoderm, and endoderm (Schoenwolf et al., 2021).

As the exact details of cellular development were not yet understood at the time that nuclear transplantation was being employed, a general consensus was nearing acceptance through the 1980s that mature embryonic cell lines were not suitable for cloning, and possibly contained genetic code dissimilar to somatic cells. The underlying mechanism of failure; however, was not impeded by the physical insertion of DNA, but rather by the misalignment of considerably imperceptible epigenomic mechanisms now deficient in the manipulated cells. To promote cellular development and a viable clone, multiple chemicals and environments were trialed, such as the media used in the foreground of cellular fusion, like caffeine, folate, and varying electric pulses (Gouveia et al., 2020).

Dolly took the world by storm in 1996 as the world's first mammal clone derived from a somatic cell of an adult organism. The new technology, termed somatic cell nuclear transfer (SCNT), was a highly volatile process involving the implantation of DNA from a mature differentiated cell into an unfertilized oocyte. A key feature of the success was the timing of the nuclear transfusion from the cell cycle of the somatic cell in relation to the enucleated oocyte. It was then realized that cell-stage incompatibility between the two cells results in greater error, namely irregular DNA replication and aneuploidy. Dolly was a groundbreaking success resulting from 277 reconstructed embryos (a yield of 0.3%) and a progeny of a mammary-gland cell (Alberio & Wolf, 2021).

Dolly developed several health complications. Soon after her surrogate delivery, it became apparent that Dolly lacked the vivacity of a similarly aged sheep. She was more frequently ill and limped at the age of five. It was first hypothesized that the endcaps of DNA, called telomeres, known to be shorter through each mitotic cycle, were causal. Extracellular variables such as ultraviolet radiation, diet, and stress were also hypothesized as factors in the degradation of DNA and premature aging. The study of the influence of these extrinsic factors on the stability of the DNA sequence has been called epigenetics. Through the years, comparative studies of environmental factors and the epigenome have yielded numerous insights about aging and multifactorial patterns of disease expression (Sinclair, 2021).

Despite the above-mentioned odds and obstacles, the origin story of SCNT has opened the door for a wide array of possibilities in trait selection, genetic engineering, and more sustainable resources. In agriculture, cloning coupled with new genetic engineering techniques has been shown to potentiate nutrient density in produce, reduce disease in livestock, and enhance growth potential. For instance, the susceptibility of tomatoes to powdery mildew-can be effectively reduced by *MLO* gene knockout. The *MILDEW RESISTANT LOCUS O (MLO)* gene is present in tomatoes and many other plants. While the molecular mechanisms of the gene are not completely understood, the *MLO* gene encodes for proteins present on the exterior of the plant cell. When the *MLO* gene is knocked out, the receptors become nonworking, and the crops become resistant to powdery mildew. Cloned crops have maintained this enhanced ability, effectively resulting in reduced food waste and increased access to fresh produce across continents (Ahmar et al., 2020). Successful techniques in animals have demonstrated similar benefits. Ultimately, however, research in SCNT has established a foundation for how cells mature, tissues are formed, and organs are made.

Scientists have long tried to find a way to harness the rejuvenating capacity of certain cells in the body. Most cells in mature organisms are differentiated, meaning they have been designated a specific job and shape. Stem cells are specialized cells that have a varying capacity to mature further into a specified role (Zakrzewski et al., 2019).

The recognition that stem cells could be used for regeneration came about in the mid 20th century following the Second World War. Secondary to research on individuals exposed to radiation, scientists became interested studying the process by which red and white blood cells were being made by the body. In studies of control mice, a reservoir of undifferentiated cells in the bone marrow, named colony-forming cells (CFUs), were discovered, which prompted multiple hypotheses on mammalian physiology. These enduring stem cells, first found by James Till and Ernest McCulloch in 1961, were used to induce hematopoiesis, the formation of differentiated blood cells, by transplanting CFUs from healthy mice into the spleens of irradiated mice (Brand-Saberi, 2020).

These studies translated well in human trials. Hematopoietic stem cell transplantation (HSCT) has shown to be clinically relevant in multiple human disorders, such as pediatric malignancy, hemoglobinopathies, and leukodystrophy. Successful treatment can be achieved in one of two ways: (1) donor stem cells are transplanted into a recipient from a genetically similar donor such as a sibling or a parent (allogeneic stem cells), or (2) transplant stem cells into a recipient harvested from their own bone marrow, umbilical cord, or other source (autologous stem cells.) Of note, in the case of blood cancers, an autologous sample would need to be obtained prior to initiation of chemotherapy. The transplanted stem cells would then repopulate in the recipient bone marrow, completely restoring the ability to form healthy blood cells across the lifetime (Brand-Saberi, 2020).

The success of HSCT and future potentially curative modalities has been hindered by the fact that the capacity of stem cells present in mature beings is limited. Stem cells have been found to have varying degrees of potency or capacity to differentiate into several cells. In humans, the liver and bone marrow contain what are called multipotent stem cells. These multipotent cells can only develop into certain types of cell lines. In bone marrow, for instance, hemopoietic cells are designed to produce various white and red blood cells. Similarly, hepatic cells have stem-cell-like properties that allow the detoxifying organ to heal or grow when damaged. Completely undifferentiated cells capable of any tissue or cell formation; however, have only been identified in the earliest embryonic stages of development (Zakrzewski et al., 2019).

In human embryos, a physiological migration of undifferentiated cells occurs in a highly ordered manner during development. These cells are grouped and located in such a way that the function of surrounding cells may turn on or off certain gene functions within the undifferentiated cell to adopt a specified role or shape. There are multiple regulatory proteins that exist in and on the outside of cells that orchestrate the activation and silencing of genes (Schoenwolf et al., 2021).

**Essential Facts**

DNA is activated by a concise interaction of proteins and molecules distributed across, in, and outside of the cell. Two key forces are (1) multiple regulatory regions that exist on DNA that help turn genes on and off, called transcription factors; and (2) exterior proteins on the surface of cells that communicate with the environment and that can activate transcription factors through a process called intracellular signaling pathways. There are numerous intracellular signaling pathways across various embryonic and adult cell types. In fetal development, intracellular signaling pathways are one process by which fetal cells are differentiated into specific cell shapes to form tissues. The pulsatory force sent from the heart, as an example, is one such trigger for Notch signaling, which sparks a cascade of brain development in neighboring cells to express proneural genes and to form differentiated neurons (Brand-Saberi, 2020).

The expanse of mechanisms that are involved in multicellular development and the epigenome have yet to be fully realized by the scientific community. Despite this, the clinical utility of such focus areas has invoked promise in the restorative possibilities and treatment of disease. To the extent of what is known about the early stages of development, animals and humans arise from a group of cells that are totipotent. Totipotency refers to the potential of a cell to form an organism. These cells next assemble into organized aggregations called germ layers and evolve to be pluripotent. Pluripotency refers to the potential to differentiate into almost any tissue or organ (with the exception of extraembryonic structures like the placenta and amnion.) Each of these cells then has the potential to form germ cells that can later differentiate into any tissue or organ (Zakrzewski et al., 2019).

Curative applications of pluripotent stem cells have been studied across multiple simple and complex organisms. In mice, for instance, healthy embryonic cells have been extracted and successfully grown in labs, where they are later transplanted into the pancreases of diabetic mice to form working islet cells (Schoenwolf et al., 2021). Despite the intent, ethical discussion surrounding human trials and similar outcomes has long been contentious within the scientific community. Once embryonic stem cells are extracted, the development potential is destroyed and the embryo is no longer viable (Brand-Saberi, 2020).

Research focused in induced pluripotent stem cells was initiated by Takahashi and Yamanaka in 2006 and helped boost the scientific inquiry on how the restorative properties of stem cells could be used.

In their work, multipotent cells were genetically reprogrammed to have pluripotent properties. Subsequent studies have found success using somatic cells (Zakrzewski et al., 2019). Studies in human iPSCs have shown promise in ophthalmologic and neurologic disease. Benefits of such an undertaking is that iPSC transplants are autologous. Thus, iPSCs have been theorized to have decreased potential of transplant rejection (Deinsberger et al., 2020).

The cost of sequencing the human genome has been steadily falling over the past 20 years since the completion of the Human Genome Project in 2003. Indeed the expense for clinical exome and genome sequencing is now covered by many insurance plans and some health systems utilize genomic sequencing as a fundamental and universal tool for all of their beneficiaries. In this age, thousands of never before recognized conditions are being discovered, and as a consequence the indications for genetic testing have been expanding (Schloss et al., 2020).

Since genes can be precisely read, or sequenced, there are multiple applications of gene editing and an array of tools that can be used to study or change a gene. Genes can be knocked out or silenced as well as corrected or added. The basic rules of gene editing comprise three overarching principles: (1) each gene contains an organized combination of sequenced nucleotides that when transcribed to RNA are then translated to form a protein; (2) double-strand breaks (DSBs) in DNA occur when DNA is cut to form a protein or when the DNA is exposed to externally caustic factors; DSBs trigger DNA repair; and (3) the naturally occurring restoration of broken or interrupted DNA is unpredictable and is accomplished by nonhomologous end joining (NHEJ) or homologous recombination (HR) (Li et al., 2020).

One of the primary challenges in the early days of gene editing was finding a way to precisely create a double stranded break. Scientists first found success with zinc-finger nucleases (ZFNs). The basic structure of ZFNs consists of a chain of proteins called zinc fingers, which function like a DNA wayfinder. The zinc fingers are constructed with transcription factors to identify three to four bases of DNA of interest. The other component is a nuclease, which will slice DNA once there is a base pair to ZFN match. Major drawbacks to ZFNs include the laborious process required in engineering a targeted DNA sequence and variable outcomes. ZFNs often do not cleave at the targeted sequence and can inadvertently cut DNA adjacent to the segment of interest. This leads to unstable DNA repair. As the double-stranded breaks brought about using ZFNs occur at an unnatural breakage point, the NHEJ process is more likely to result in randomized nucleotide insertion or deletion at the breakage point. This can then result in either a reduction or termination in the functionality of a gene. As a useful application, ZFNs have allowed scientists to create knockdown and knockout animal models to study how a gene works (Khalil, 2020).

Clustered Regularly Interspaced Short Palindromic Repeats (CRISPR) and associated proteins make for one of the most versatile gene-editing technologies being used today. To abridge the process, a DNA transport vehicle called Cas-9 nuclease, a naturally occurring protective enzyme found within bacteria, is commandeered to target and change a specific sequence or gene. The complex is normally activated in bacteria when viral DNA is inserted into the cell. Portions of the invading viral DNA are cleaved by the Cas-9 nuclease and stored in the bacterial DNA for future attacks. Should the virus invade the bacteria again, the CAS-9 system will latch on to the recognized RNA segments and use a key called a protospacer adjacent motif (PAM) to recognize nonbacterial DNA and cleave the viral DNA (Li et al., 2020).

In a lab, the CRISPR-Cas9 system uses the bacterial enzyme Cas-9 nuclease and other similar enzymatic species in an isolated form. The enzyme is then introduced to a segment of information called single-guide RNA (sgRNA). sgRNA is engineered in a lab to contain a specific sequence of palindromic nucleotides and will correspond with a genomic sequence of interest. The conjoined system of Cas-9 and sgRNA is then fed an additional section of instructions in the form of a protospacer adjacent motif (PAM) that will function like an anchor to a corresponding DNA target site where a double stranded break will be made. When the tailored Cas-9 enzyme is later introduced to cellular DNA with nucleotides corresponding to the sgRNA, the PAM site latches to the DNA and generates DSBs. In the absence of guide RNA, the gene may be knocked out or knocked down. If the sgRNA within the CAS-9 system, however, contains working sgRNA nucleotides, then homology-directed repair (HDR) can occur, as opposed to the naturally occurring NHEJ repair pathway, and can result in a functional gene (Li et al., 2020).

## VIGNETTE

Pearl S. Buck has expressed her desire for genomic treatment and cure in her Pulitzer Prize winning book, *The Good Earth*. Her deep empathy for humankind was likely inspired by her own child, Carol Buck, born in 1920, and to Carol's devastating cognitive decline as a result of Phenylalanine hydroxylase (PAH) deficiency, an inborn error of metabolism that had not been discovered in those times (Finger & Christ, 2004). Asbjørn Følling, a Norwegian doctor and biochemist, would not discover phenylpyruvic acid in urine as a sign and early manifestation of the genetic disorder until 1935. A more efficient process to screen for this treatable disorder by way of a bacterial inhibition assay was then devised by Dr. Robert Guthrie in 1958. Early detection of PAH deficiency in infants gave way to treatment. Treated infants grew to have normal intelligence through adulthood. Given the success and improved capability to screen for a broader panel of treatable genetic disorders, Newborn Screening (NBS) was then implemented for all babies born in the United States through the 1960s (Vill et al., 2019).

Beginning in 2008, NBS expanded from testing only biochemical analytes to testing DNA extracted from NBS spot cards. This allowed for the expansion of screening for genetic disorders. Spinal Muscular Atrophy (SMA) is one such disorder recently added to the Recommended Uniform Screening Panel (RUSP) in 2018. *SMN1*-related spinal muscular atrophy (SMA) is a variably expressed condition caused by degeneration of the anterior horn cells in the spinal cord. The disorder is characterized by progressive muscle weakness and respiratory insufficiency leading to paralysis and death (Woener et al., 2021). Onasemnogene abeparvovec (Zolgensma) was approved by the U.S. Food and Drug Administration for the treatment of pediatric patients less than 2 years of age with SMA on May 24, 2019. Unlike its predecessors, Zolgensma is not a metabolic food product, medication, hormone, or supplement. It is a gene replacement therapy. Zolgensma is administered as a one time intravenous infusion and works by replacing the nonworking *SMN1* gene in infants and children with SMA type 1 with a working copy of the gene (Mercuri et al., 2021).

## END-OF-CHAPTER QUESTIONS

1. What is the epigenome?
2. What is a pluripotent stem cell?
3. How are DNA breakage points normally repaired?
4. What is the purpose of single-guide RNA (sgRNA)?

## REFERENCES

Ahmar, S., Gill, R. A., Jung, K. H., Faheem, A., Qasim, M. U., Mubeen, M., & Zhou, W. (2020). Conventional and molecular techniques from simple breeding to speed breeding in crop plants: Recent advances and future outlook. *International Journal of Molecular Sciences, 21*(7), 2590. https://doi.org/10.3390/ijms21072590

Alberio, R., & Wolf, E. (2021). 25th anniversary of cloning by somatic-cell nuclear transfer: Nuclear transfer and the development of genetically modified/gene edited livestock. *Reproduction, 162*(1), F59–F68. https://doi.org/10.1530/REP-21-0078

Brand-Saberi, B. (2020). *Essential current concepts in stem cell biology* (1st ed.). Springer International Publishing.

Deinsberger, J., Reisinger, D., & Weber, B. (2020). Global trends in clinical trials involving pluripotent stem cells: A systematic multi-database analysis. npj Regenerative Medicin, *5*, 15. https://doi.org/10.1038/s41536-020-00100-4

Finger, S., & Christ, S. E. (2004). Pearl S. Buck and Phenylketonuria (PKU). *Journal of the History of the Neurosciences, 13*(1), 44–57. https://doi.org/10.1080/09647040490885484

Gouveia, C., Carin, H., Egli, D., & Pepper, M. S. (2020). Lessons learned from somatic cell nuclear transfer. *International Journal of Molecular Sciences, 21*(7), 2314. https://doi.org/10.3390/ijms21072314

Khalil, A. M. (2020). The genome editing revolution: review. *Journal, Genetic Engineering & Biotechnology, 18*(1), 68. https://doi.org/10.1186/s43141-020-00078-y

Li, H., Yang, Y., Hong, W., Huang, M., Wu, M., & Zhao, X. (2020). Applications of genome editing technology in the targeted therapy of human diseases: Mechanisms, advances and prospects. *Signal Transduction and Targeted Therapy, 5*, 1. https://doi.org/10.1038/s41392-019-0089-y

Mercuri, E., Muntoni, F., Baranello, G., Masson, R., Boespflug-Tanguy, O., Bruno, C., Corti, S., Daron, A., Deconinck, N., Servais, L., Straub, V., Ouyang, H., Chand, D., Tauscher-Wisniewski, S., Mendonca, N., Lavrov, A., Seferian, A., De Lucia, S., Tachibana, S., … Brolatti, N. (2021). Onasemnogene abeparvovec gene therapy for symptomatic infantile-onset spinal muscular atrophy type 1 (STR1VE-EU): An open-label, single-arm, multicentre, phase 3 trial. *Lancet Neurology, 20*(10), 832–841. https://doi.org/10.1016/S1474-4422(21)00251-9

Schloss, Gibbs, R. A., Makhijani, V. B., & Marziali, A. (2020). Cultivating DNA Sequencing Technology After the Human Genome Project. *Annual Review of Genomics and Human Genetics, 21*(1), 117–138. https://doi.org/10.1146/annurev-genom-111919-082433

Schoenwolf, G. C., Bleyl, S. B., Brauer, P. R., Francis-West, P. H., & Larsen, W. J. (2021). *Larsen's human embryology* (6th ed.). Elsevier.

Simmet, K., Wolf, E., & Zakhartchenko, V. (2021). Manipulating the epigenome in nuclear transfer cloning: Where, when and how. *International Journal of Molecular Sciences, 22*(1), 236. https://doi.org/10.3390/ijms22010236

Sinclair, K. D. (2021). Dolly at 25 . . . is she '. . . still goin' strong?' *Reproduction, 162*(1), E1–E3. https://doi.org/10.1530/REP-21-0212

Takahashi, K., Yamanaka, S. (2006). Induction of pluripotent stem cells from mouse embryonic and adult fibroblast cultures by defined factors. *Cell. 126*(4):663–76. doi: 10.1016/j.cell.2006.07.024. Epub 2006 Aug 10.

Vill, K., Kölbel, H., Schwartz, O., Blaschek, A., Olgemöller, B., Harms, E., Burggraf, S., Röschinger, W., Durner, J., Gläser, D., Nennstiel, U., Wirth, B., Schara, U., Jensen, B., Becker, M., Hohenfellner, K., & Müller-Felber, W. (2019). One year of newborn screening for SMA — Results of a

German pilot project. *Journal of Neuromuscular Diseases*, *6*(4), 503–515. https://doi.org/10.3233/JND-190428

Woerner, A. C., Gallagher, R. C., Vockley, J., & Adhikari, A. N. (2021). The use of whole genome and exome sequencing for newborn screening: Challenges and opportunities for population health. *Frontiers in Pediatrics*, *9*, 663752. https://doi.org/10.3389/fped.2021.663752

Zakrzewski, W., Dobrzyński, M., Szymonowicz, M., & Rybak, Z. (2019) Stem cells: Past, present, and future. *Stem Cell Research & Therapy*, *10*(1), 68. https://doi.org/10.1186/s13287-019-1165-5

# 15

# Genomics in Healthcare

Kathleen A. Calzone

*The integration of genomics into healthcare has expanded exponentially, in part due to the substantial reduction in genomics sequencing costs, from $100,000,000 in 2001 to less than $1,000 in 2021 (National Human Genome Research Institute, 2021). These costs are similar to costs for other medical tests that enable genomic technology and resulting information to be integrated into routine healthcare. Evidence-based clinical applications of genomics now span the entire healthcare continuum from before birth to after death. This chapter provides a brief overview of the current landscape of genomic clinical applications, the ongoing integration of precision health, and the essential elements needed for the implementation of precision health and genomics into a practice.*

**In this chapter, you will learn:**

1. To explain the applications of genomics in healthcare across the life continuum
2. To discuss the intersection between genomics and precision health
3. To identify the critical components of integrating precision health and genomics into healthcare
4. To summarize the resources available for the integration of precision health and genomics

## GENOMIC APPLICATIONS TO HEALTHCARE ACROSS THE LIFE CONTINUUM

Genomics has evidence-based clinical applications that span the entire healthcare continuum from before birth to after death (Table 15.1). Despite the expanding evidence-based genomic

Table 15.1

**Clinical Applications**

| Life Continuum | Example Genomic Evidence-Based Clinical Applications |
|---|---|
| Preconception | Genetic testing for carrier status prior to pregnancy, often for autosomal recessive disorders such as sickle cell disease, cystic fibrosis, or MUTYH-associated polyposis (MAP) (Committee Opinion No. 690: Carrier Screening in the Age of Genomic Medicine, 2017).<br>Predisposition genomic testing using chorionic villus sampling and amniocentesis using preimplantation genomic diagnosis in individuals with a known pathogenic variant to avoid genetic transmission of the variant (Dahdouh et al., 2015). |
| Prenatal | Noninvasive prenatal screening using cell-free fetal DNA testing in women with a clinical indication such as advanced maternal age (Allyse et al., 2015; Sabbagh & Van den Veyver, 2020). |
| Newborn Screening | Public health approach to the identification and management of health conditions identifiable in the newborn where early intervention could result in improved outcomes. Conducted using a dried blood spot from a heel prick. Results can indicate a need for a genomic evaluation (Martiniano et al., 2021).<br>Research is ongoing assessing the utility of whole genome or whole exome sequencing in newborns (Woerner et al., 2021).<br>Residual dried blood-spot cards can be stored for future research as they are a source of genomic information (Sok et al., 2020). |
| Risk Identification | Genomic testing for variants in disease predisposition genes associated with a wide range of diseases such as cancer and cardiovascular conditions (Cirino et al., 2017; Grant et al., 2021; Whitworth et al., 2018).<br>Single-nucleotide polymorphism (SNP) tests to increase the precision of risk calculations using polygenic risk scores (Slunecka et al., 2021). |

(*continued*)

Table 15.1

**Clinical Applications (*continued*)**

| Life Continuum | Example Genomic Evidence-Based Clinical Applications |
|---|---|
| Screening and Diagnosis | Screening tests that include DNA analysis such as the multitarget stool DNA test, a less-invasive genomic test to screen for colon polyps or cancer (Bosch et al., 2019). |
| Disease Characterization | Somatic testing for genomic variants that can inform prognosis and potentially therapeutic decision-making such as in melanoma (Wróblewska et al., 2021). |
| Individualized Therapy | Somatic genomic testing in cancer to identify candidates for molecularly targeted therapies (Hicks et al., 2021). Preemptive pharmacogenomic testing to inform medication selection and/or dosing (David et al., 2021). |
| Symptom Management | Priority area of research is the study of the genomic influences of symptoms and symptom clusters (Singh et al., 2020). |
| After Death | Use of stored specimens for posthumous genomic testing for familial information (Bilkey et al., 2019). Use of stored specimens for research purposes (Tassé, 2011). |

applications, there is ample evidence that nursing has limited genomic capacity. This includes studies documenting that faculty who are training new nurses or those pursuing advanced degrees have a knowledge base equivalent to that of the students they teach (Donnelly et al., 2017; Read & Ward, 2016, 2018). In practice, multiple studies have demonstrated deficits in practicing-nurse genomic capacity, with little improvement seen in the past several years (Wright et al., 2018).

Reasons for this sustained deficit in nursing genomic capacity are considered to be because genomics represents a complex competency. Nursing has no scientific knowledge base in genomics upon which to build upon. This differs from other change initiatives, such as the COVID-19 pandemic, where all nursing had a foundation in core infectious disease principles that allowed them to quickly pivot their practice. Faculty and continuing educators have limited capacity to teach genomic information. And the availability of clinical placements where genomics is being used by nurses can be limited. This is complicated further because many genomic applications are not observable. Consider pharmacogenomics, where based on a genomic test the correct medication at the correct dose was ordered, resulting in the expected efficacy and limited toxicity. Contrast this to pain, where an intervention is implemented to ameliorate that pain, which can be readily observable. The pharmacogenomic example requires the nurse to have an underpinning in the genomics of drug metabolism to appreciate why the outcome was achieved. The language of genomics is also not well understood , thus hampering the ability of nurses and nursing faculty to read the literature. Lastly, this requires leadership to have sufficient genomic competency to recognize the value of supporting genomic education initiatives (Calzone, 2018b).

## PRECISION HEALTH AND GENOMICS

The rapidly expanding genomic evidence base coupled with advances in technology has resulted in a transition from a focus on single genes (genetics) into genomics, the full complement of genomic cellular instructions (Consensus Panel on Genetic/Genomic Nursing Competencies, 2009). However, genomics does not work in isolation and is influenced by the environment, including psychosocial, cultural factors, lifestyle, behaviors, and economics, which is the essence of precision health (Fu et al., 2020). Together, precision health and genomics have been found to improve therapeutic efficacy, improve the safety and quality of healthcare, and reduce healthcare costs, which is especially relevant in common complex health conditions such as cancer (Weymann et al., 2021). The clinical relevance of precision health and genomics spans the entire healthcare continuum (Franks et al., 2021).

Therefore, all nurses, regardless of their role, practice setting, academic training, or clinical and/or population specialty, must have a sufficient foundation in precision health and genomics. To guide capacity building in genomics, nursing competencies that were both foundational (which include knowledge elements and clinical performance indicators) and then leveled for advanced practice were developed in the United States, as well as in a few other countries (Calzone et al., 2018a; Consensus Panel on Genetic/Genomic Nursing Competencies, 2009; Greco et al., 2012). In the United States these competencies are actively being updated. At the doctoral level the Genomic Knowledge Matrix was established to guide capacity building based on the role an individual plays in nursing science (Regan et al., 2019). Lastly, there is an ongoing initiative by the Global Genomics Nursing Alliance (G2NA) to establish global minimal genomic competencies and competencies specific to precision health.

## INTEGRATION OF PRECISION HEALTH AND GENOMICS IN PRACTICE

Precision health and genomic clinical applications can benefit from infrastructure that facilitates their integration into practice. Importantly, nursing as well as other healthcare providers could benefit from point-of-care decision support tools being integrated into the electronic health record. Consider that currently there are 26 Clinical Pharmacogenomic Implementation Consortium (CPIC) guidelines that cover evidence-based pharmacogenomic applications for more than 160 commonly prescribed medications (Clinical Pharmacogenetics Implementation Consortium, 2021). Additionally, support tools can include the ability to document and update at each encounter family history in the form of a pedigree, and an established location to find genomic testing reports in an electronic health record, as many tests are performed by outside vendors and reports can be buried in outside records. Additionally, nurses need access to clinical resources leveled for nursing. Most important, access to genomic experts varies based on the setting, so nurses may not have someone to go to for help. Healthcare settings need to consider how to provide this level of consultation support. Healthcare leadership must have an adequate understanding of the complexity of genomics to establish mechanisms to support nurses and other healthcare professions in the integration of precision health and genomics (Calzone, 2018b).

## RESOURCES FOR THE INTEGRATION OF PRECISION HEALTH GENOMICS

Globally, the integration of genomics into nursing education and practice is very uneven, driven largely by the complexity of the information and the lack of an underpinning in genomics and precision health. Implementation efforts, whether in education or practice environments, therefore can benefit from detailed guidance. The G2NA established a maturity matrix that provides a means to assess where you are in the implementation pathway, identify areas for improvement, guide interventions, and measure progress over time (Tonkin et al., 2020a). This instrument, Assessment of Strategic Integration of Genomics Across Nursing (ASIGN), is based on the identification of six critical success factors. Each critical success factor has established key enablers to guide users and are evaluated based on five stages of maturity that range from precontemplation to leading (Tonkin et al., 2020a). Supplementing ASIGN is a detailed road map designed to facilitate operationalizing an implementation plan.

**Essential Facts**

**Critical Success Factors**

1. Enhanced education and workforce development
2. Effective nursing practice
3. Infrastructure and resources that support incorporation of genomics in practice
4. Interprofessional collaboration and communication
5. Family- and community-focused care
6. Healthcare transformed through policy and leadership

### Road Map Implementation Stages

Figure 15.1 provides guidance on the elements that can facilitate integration initiatives as guided by the Consolidated Framework for Implementation Research, which integrates the critical elements from 19 theoretical frameworks to optimize implementation research (Damschroder et al., 2009; Tonkin et al., 2020b). Together, the road map and ASIGN provide the guidance needed to facilitate precision health and genomic integration in any clinical or academic setting.

**Figure 15.1** Road map implementation stages.

## END-OF-CHAPTER QUESTIONS

1. From the list below, select the evidence-based clinical applications of genomics currently available in practice. (Select all that apply.)
   - Preconception genomic testing
   - Pharmacogenomic testing
   - Somatic testing
   - Cardiovascular predisposition genomic testing

- None of the above
- All of the above

2. What are the elements of precision health?
   - Pharmacogenomic testing
   - Integration of information on genomics, environment, personal and lifestyle factors, culture, and the environment to inform healthcare decision-making
   - Molecularly targeted therapy
   - Predisposition genetic testing
3. Which of the following are critical success factors associated with the integration of precision health and genomics?
   - Enhanced education and workforce development
   - Nurses certified in genomics
   - Infrastructure and resources that support incorporation of genomics in practice
   - Genomic testing availability
4. Do all nurses have genomic competencies to guide education and practice?
   - Yes
   - No
   - Not sure

## VIGNETTE

There are currently more than 76,000 genomic tests for over 10,000 health conditions (Genetic Testing Registry, 2021). However, many of these tests are not used despite evidence-based guidelines. Consider the case of a male in his 70s with lower extremity vascular disease undergoing bypass surgery. IV morphine was ordered for postoperative pain control in the recovery room. The patient reported no relief from his pain through the use of morphine, so he was administered additional doses and continued to report no relief. He ultimately developed respiratory depression, required resuscitation, and was transferred to the intensive care unit (ICU). For subsequent surgeries to address his lower extremity vascular disease, the postoperative course in the recovery room was complicated by lack of pain control using morphine, resulting in repeat episodes of respiratory depression and transfers into the ICU.

***Were these events preventable?*** Yes, the phenotype of an individual receiving no pain relief at all from the prescribed medication was an indication that this patient may have a variant in a drug-metabolizing gene affecting morphine metabolism. The phenotype should have been recognized by the recovery nurse caring for the patient who should have contacted the ordering provider to modify the postoperative pain control order.

***Was pharmacogenomic testing indicated for this patient?*** Pharmacogenomic testing may have benefited the patient but recognizing the phenotype alone should have been sufficient. However, a sufficient underpinning in pharmacogenomics is required to recognize the phenotype.

***Did this episode affect the quality and safety of the healthcare delivered to this patient?*** Yes, this was life threatening and prolonged the patient's recovery.

***What were the other impacts associated with these episodes?*** This drastically increased the healthcare costs for the patient and his family. Additionally, this increased the distress on the family. The postoperative recovery was extended, including his hospital stay.

***Could these episodes have been avoided?*** Yes, preemptive pharmacogenomic testing could have informed optimal pain control medication selection and dosing which is the essence of precision health and genomics. Even in the absence of a pharmacogenomic test, recognition of the phenotype by the healthcare providers could have resulted in a different outcome. Additionally, all providers need to recognize that the one-size-fits-all approach may be easier but increases healthcare costs and decreases quality and safety.

In summary, precision health and genomics requires a prepared workforce and can benefit from point-of-care support. Testing technology has drastically decreased in cost, but with healthcare providers who have a sufficient underpinning in precision health and genomics, testing may not always be required if the phenotype can be recognized and addressed. In summary, the integration of precision health and genomics across all of healthcare has the potential to improve both the quality and safety of healthcare and health outcomes.

## REFERENCES

Allyse, M., Minear, M. A., Berson, E., Sridhar, S., Rote, M., Hung, A., & Chandrasekharan, S. (2015). Non-invasive prenatal testing: A review of international implementation and challenges. *International Journal of Women's Health*, *7*, 113–126. https://doi.org/10.2147/ijwh.S67124

Bilkey, G. A., Burns, B. L., Coles, E. P., Bowman, F. L., Beilby, J. P., Pachter, N. S., Baynam, G., Dawkins, H. J. S., Nowak, K. J., & Weeramanthri, T. S. (2019). Genomic testing for human health and disease across the life cycle: Applications and ethical, legal, and social challenges. *Frontiers in Public Health*, *7*, 40. https://doi.org/10.3389/fpubh.2019.00040

Bosch, L. J. W., Melotte, V., Mongera, S., Daenen, K. L. J., Coupé, V. M. H., van Turenhout, S. T., Stoop, E. M., de Wijkerslooth, T. R., Mulder, C. J. J., Rausch, C., Kuipers, E. J., Dekker, E., Domanico, M. J., Lidgard, G. P., Berger, B. M., van Engeland, M., Carvalho, B., & Meijer, G. A. (2019). Multitarget stool DNA test performance in an average-risk colorectal cancer screening population. *American Journal of Gastroenterology, 114*(12), 1909–1918. https://doi.org/10.14309/ajg.0000000000000445

Calzone, K. A., Kirk, M., Tonkin, E., Badzek, L., Benjamin, C., & Middleton, A. (2018a). Increasing nursing capacity in genomics: Overview of existing global genomics resources. *Nurse Education Today, 69*, 53–59. https://doi.org/10.1016/j.nedt.2018.06.032

Calzone, K., Jenkins, J., Culp, S., & Badzek, L. (2018b). Hospital nursing leadership led interventions increased genomic awareness and educational intent in Magnet® settings. *Nursing Outlook, 66*(3), 244–253.

Cirino, A. L., Harris, S., Lakdawala, N. K., Michels, M., Olivotto, I., Day, S. M., Abrams, D. J., Charron, P., Caleshu, C., Semsarian, C., Ingles, J., Rakowski, H., Judge, D. P., & Ho, C. Y. (2017). Role of genetic testing in inherited cardiovascular disease: A review. *JAMA Cardiology, 2*(10), 1153–1160. https://doi.org/10.1001/jamacardio.2017.2352

Clinical Pharmacogenetics Implementation Consortium. (2021). Clinical Pharmacogenetics Implementation Consortium. Retrieved September 24, 2021, from https://cpicpgx.org/

Committee Opinion No. 690: Carrier Screening in the Age of Genomic Medicine. (2017). *Obstetrics & Gynecology, 129*(3), e35–e40. https://doi.org/10.1097/aog.0000000000001951

Consensus Panel on Genetic/Genomic Nursing Competencies. (2009). *Essentials of genetic and genomic nursing: Competencies, curricula guidelines, and outcome indicators* (2nd ed.). American Nurses Association.

Dahdouh, E. M., Balayla, J., Audibert, F., Wilson, R. D., Audibert, F., Brock, J. A., Campagnolo, C., Carroll, J., Chong, K., Gagnon, A., Johnson, J. A., MacDonald, W., Okun, N., Pastuck, M., & Vallée-Pouliot, K. (2015). Technical update: Preimplantation genetic diagnosis and screening. *Journal of Obstetrics and Gynaecology Canada, 37*(5), 451–463. https://doi.org/10.1016/s1701-2163(15)30261-9

Damschroder, L. J., Aron, D. C., Keith, R. E., Kirsh, S. R., Alexander, J. A., & Lowery, J. C. (2009). Fostering implementation of health services research findings into practice: a consolidated framework for advancing implementation science. *Implementation Science, 4*, 50. https://doi.org/10.1186/1748-5908-4-50

David, V., Fylan, B., Bryant, E., Smith, H., Sagoo, G. S., & Rattray, M. (2021). An analysis of pharmacogenomic-guided pathways and their effect on medication changes and hospital admissions: A systematic review and meta-analysis. *Frontiers in Genetics, 12*, 698148. https://doi.org/10.3389/fgene.2021.698148

Donnelly, M. K., Nersesian, P. V., Foronda, C., Jones, E. L., & Belcher, A. E. (2017). Nurse faculty knowledge of and confidence in teaching genetics/genomics: Implications for faculty development. *Nurse Education, 42*(2), 100–104. https://doi.org/10.1097/nne.0000000000000297

Franks, P. W., Melén, E., Friedman, M., Sundström, J., Kockum, I., Klareskog, L., Almqvist, C., Bergen, S. E., Czene, K., Hägg, S., Hall, P., Johnell, K., Malarstig, A., Catrina, A., Hagström, H., Benson, M., Gustav Smith, J., Gomez, M. F., Orho-Melander, M., … Sullivan, P. F. (2021). Technological readiness and implementation of genomic-driven precision medicine for complex diseases. *Journal of Internal Medicine*, *290*(3), 602–620. https://doi.org/10.1111/joim.13330

Fu, M. R., Kurnat-Thoma, E., Starkweather, A., Henderson, W. A., Cashion, A. K., Williams, J. K., Katapodi, M. C., Reuter-Rice, K., Hickey, K. T., Barcelona de Mendoza, V., Calzone, K., Conley, Y. P., Anderson, C. M., Lyon, D. E., Weaver, M. T., Shiao, P. K., Constantino, R. E., Wung, S. F., Hammer, M. J., … Coleman, B. (2020). Precision health: A nursing perspective. *International Journal of Nursing Sciences*, *7*(1), 5–12. https://doi.org/10.1016/j.ijnss.2019.12.008

Genetic Testing Registry. (2021). GTR data. Retrieved September 20, 2021, from https://www.ncbi.nlm.nih.gov/gtr/

Grant, C. N., Rhee, D., Tracy, E. T., Aldrink, J. H., Baertschiger, R. M., Lautz, T. B., Glick, R. D., Rodeberg, D. A., Ehrlich, P. F., & Christison-Lagay, E. (2021). Pediatric solid tumors and associated cancer predisposition syndromes: Workup, management, and surveillance. A summary from the APSA cancer committee. *Journal of Pediatric Surgery*. https://doi.org/10.1016/j.jpedsurg.2021.08.008

Greco, K. E., Tinley, S., & Seibert, D. (2012). *Essential genetic and genomic competencies for nurses with graduate degrees*. American Nurses Association. Retrieved May 22, 2012, from http://www.nursingworld.org/MainMenuCategories/EthicsStandards/Genetics-1/Essential-Genetic-and-Genomic-Competencies-for-Nurses-With-Graduate-Degrees.pdf

Hicks, J. K., Howard, R., Reisman, P., Adashek, J. J., Fields, K. K., Gray, J. E., McIver, B., McKee, K., O'Leary, M. F., Perkins, R. M., Robinson, E., Tandon, A., Teer, J. K., Markowitz, J., & Rollison, D. E. (2021). Integrating somatic and germline next-generation sequencing into routine clinical oncology practice. *JCO Precision Oncology*, *5*. https://doi.org/10.1200/po.20.00513

Martiniano, S. L., Elbert, A. A., Farrell, P. M., Ren, C. L., Sontag, M. K., Wu, R., & McColley, S. A. (2021). Outcomes of infants born during the first 9 years of CF newborn screening in the United States: A retrospective Cystic Fibrosis Foundation Patient Registry cohort study. *Pediatric Pulmonology*, *56*, 3758–3767. https://doi.org/10.1002/ppul.25658

National Human Genome Research Institute. (2021). *DNA sequencing costs: Data*. Retrieved September 28, 2021, from https://www.genome.gov/about-genomics/fact-sheets/DNA-Sequencing-Costs-Data

Read, C. Y., & Ward, L. D. (2016). Faculty performance on the genomic nursing concept inventory. *Journal of Nursing Scholarship*, *48*(1), 5–13. https://doi.org/10.1111/jnu.12175

Read, C. Y., & Ward, L. D. (2018). Misconceptions about genomics among nursing faculty and students. *Nurse Educator*, *43*(4), 196–200. https://doi.org/10.1097/nne.0000000000000444

Regan, M., Engler, M. B., Coleman, B., Daack-Hirsch, S., & Calzone, K. A. (2019). Establishing the genomic knowledge matrix for nursing science. *Journal of Nursing Scholarship, 51*(1), 50–57. https://doi.org/10.1111/jnu.12427

Sabbagh, R., & Van den Veyver, I. B. (2020). The current and future impact of genome-wide sequencing on fetal precision medicine. *Human Genetics, 139*(9), 1121–1130. https://doi.org/10.1007/s00439-019-02088-4

Singh, K. P., Dhruva, A., Flowers, E., Paul, S. M., Hammer, M. J., Wright, F., Cartwright, F., Conley, Y. P., Melisko, M., Levine, J. D., Miaskowski, C., & Kober, K. M. (2020). Alterations in patterns of gene expression and perturbed pathways in the gut-brain axis are associated with chemotherapy-induced nausea. *Journal of Pain and Symptom Management, 59*(6), 1248–1259.e1245. https://doi.org/10.1016/j.jpainsymman.2019.12.352

Slunecka, J. L., van der Zee, M. D., Beck, J. J., Johnson, B. N., Finnicum, C. T., Pool, R., Hottenga, J. J., de Geus, E. J. C., & Ehli, E. A. (2021). Implementation and implications for polygenic risk scores in healthcare. *Human Genomics, 15*(1), 46. https://doi.org/10.1186/s40246-021-00339-y

Sok, P., Lupo, P. J., Richard, M. A., Rabin, K. R., Ehli, E. A., Kallsen, N. A., Davies, G. E., Scheurer, M. E., & Brown, A. L. (2020). Utilization of archived neonatal dried blood spots for genome-wide genotyping. *PLoS One, 15*(2), e0229352. https://doi.org/10.1371/journal.pone.0229352

Tassé, A. M. (2011). Biobanking and deceased persons. *Human Genetics, 130*(3), 415–423. https://doi.org/10.1007/s00439-011-1049-y

Tonkin, E., Calzone, K. A., Badzek, L., Benjamin, C., Middleton, A., Patch, C., & Kirk, M. (2020a). A maturity matrix for nurse leaders to facilitate and benchmark progress in genomic healthcare policy, infrastructure, education, and delivery. *Journal of Nursing Scholarship, 52*(5), 583–592. https://doi.org/10.1111/jnu.12586

Tonkin, E., Calzone, K. A., Badzek, L., Benjamin, C., Middleton, A., Patch, C., & Kirk, M. (2020b). A roadmap for global acceleration of genomics integration across nursing. *Journal of Nursing Scholarship, 52*(3), 329–338. https://doi.org/10.1111/jnu.12552

Weymann, D., Pollard, S., Chan, B., Titmuss, E., Bohm, A., Laskin, J., Jones, S. J. M., Pleasance, E., Nelson, J., Fok, A., Lim, H., Karsan, A., Renouf, D. J., Schrader, K. A., Sun, S., Yip, S., Schaeffer, D. F., Marra, M. A., & Regier, D. A. (2021). Clinical and cost outcomes following genomics-informed treatment for advanced cancers. *Cancer Medicine, 10*(15), 5131–5140. https://doi.org/10.1002/cam4.4076

Whitworth, J., Smith, P. S., Martin, J. E., West, H., Luchetti, A., Rodger, F., Clark, G., Carss, K., Stephens, J., Stirrups, K., Penkett, C., Mapeta, R., Ashford, S., Megy, K., Shakeel, H., Ahmed, M., Adlard, J., Barwell, J., Brewer, C., … Maher, E. R. (2018). Comprehensive cancer-predisposition gene testing in an adult multiple primary tumor series shows a broad range of deleterious variants and atypical tumor phenotypes. *American Journal of Human Genetics, 103*(1), 3–18. https://doi.org/10.1016/j.ajhg.2018.04.013

Woerner, A. C., Gallagher, R. C., Vockley, J., & Adhikari, A. N. (2021). The use of whole genome and exome sequencing for newborn screening: Challenges and opportunities for population health. *Frontiers in Pediatrics*, *9*, 663752. https://doi.org/10.3389/fped.2021.663752

Wright, H., Zhao, L., Birks, M., & Mills, J. (2018). Nurses' competence in genetics: An integrative review. *Nursing & Health Sciences*, *20*(2), 142–153. https://doi.org/10.1111/nhs.12401

Wróblewska, J. P., Dias-Santagata, D., Ustaszewski, A., Wu, C. L., Fujimoto, M., Selim, M. A., Biernat, W., Ryś, J., Marszalek, A., & Hoang, M. P. (2021). Prognostic roles of BRAF, KIT, NRAS, IGF2R and SF3B1 mutations in mucosal melanomas. *Cells*, *10*(9), 2216. https://doi.org/10.3390/cells10092216

# 16

# Answers to End-of-Chapter Questions

## CHAPTER 1: INTRODUCTION TO GENETICS AND GENOMICS

1. The Human Genome project improved the diagnosis of genetic disorders, increased the technology available to sequence the genome, and shared important genomic data across the globe.
2. There are thousands of conditions that can be chosen for this answer. From the section, cystic fibrosis is a Mendelian condition caused by a single-gene mutation. Depression, for example, is a multifactorial condition caused by genetics, family history, and an individual's environment.
3. Nucleotide base pairs, gene, DNA, chromosome, genome.
4. E. All of the above.

## CHAPTER 2: GENE EXPRESSION

1. Genotype is the combination of alleles a person has. Phenotype is the observable effect exerted by those alleles.
2. There are many differences between DNA and RNA, but two of the clearest are that RNA is single stranded and uses the letters A, C, U, and G. DNA is double stranded and uses A, C, T, and G.
3. Transcription is the process by which RNA is produced using DNA as a template. Translation is the process by which protein is synthesized from RNA.

4. While both are functional parts of a gene, exons are the protein-coding regions of the gene, while introns carry instructions for where, when, and how much of the gene should be expressed.
5. Our genes can be spliced in many ways, sometimes including specific exons, sometimes omitting others. Since the protein-coding exons included in the final instructions for the protein are different, the protein itself will be different too. In this way, the same gene can produce different proteins.
6. Certain environmental exposures can alter methylation patterns, causing certain genes to become hyper- or hypomethylated. This will, in turn, alter the expression of those genes.
7. While there are many others, two major epigenetic methods our bodies use to control gene expression are methylation and histone modification.

## CHAPTER 3: MEDICAL FAMILY HISTORY

- Adoption
  - Information about the adoptive family's health, social, and environmental exposures can help sort out health risk that are not genetic. However, inherited genetic risk cannot be discerned from the adoptive family.
- Cultural definitions of family
  - Extended family members can be referred to differently depending on cultural definitions associated with terms like cousin, aunt and uncle. Terms like "second cousin" and "once removed" are often misunderstood and applied inconsistently. The degree of relationship is important to know when calculating genetic risk. Depicting the relationships in a pedigree rather than relying on oral reporting can define the degree of relationship among family members more accurately.
- Cultural biases
  - Some degrees of consanguinity are more or less culturally acceptable and differ among people. It is important to identify consanguineous relationships because these can increase genetic risk for recessive disorders. Avoiding the topic because you are uncomfortable could fail to identify increased risk due to consanguinity. Some people can falsely assume that disorders are more or less prevalent in a population. Provider biases may lead to under ascertainment of the phenotype. Patient biases may lead to under-reporting of phenotype.

- Misattributed paternity
  - Misattributed paternity falsely assumes the biological identify of a parent and can lead to under or over estimation of genetic risk.
- Non-traditional families
  - While all relationships within a family contribute to the health and wellbeing of the family members, it is important to clarify biological relationships to determine inherited genetic risk.
- Reliability of information
  - In order for the family medical history to be useful it must be accurate. Some family members are better historians than others. Allowing time for patients to collect information from multiple family sources and to obtain medical records to validate health information are strategies to enhance the reliability of the information.

## CHAPTER 5: CANCER GENETICS: WHEN A GOOD CELL BEHAVES BADLY

1. The cell synthesizes the DNA in the S phase of the cell cycle.
2. Common chromosome abnormalities in cancer cells include deletions and duplications.
3. The transformation step is where the cell has progressed to a precancerous cell.
4. A tumor suppressor gene acts as a "brake" on cell division and tumor development.
5. A double-strand DNA break is devastating to a cell and is utilized in radiation therapy for cancer.
6. Over 90% of cancer deaths are caused by metastasis.
7. The NER pathway repairs sunlight-induced DNA damage.
8. The two arms of the immune system are the innate and adaptive systems.
9. The T-cell is the first line of protection from pathogens and tumor cells.
10. Approximately 5% to 10% of patients who develop cancer have an inherited cancer predisposition syndrome.
11. There are many cancer predisposition syndromes: Lynch syndrome, the breast/ovarian cancer syndromes (*BRCA1* & *2*), Li-Fraumeni syndrome, and others.
12. The chemical weapons used in World Wars I and II that led to the development of the first chemotherapy agents were the sulfur mustard gases.
13. Rituximab was the first monoclonal antibody therapeutic agent.
14. Pembrolizumab blocks the PD-1 pathway.

## CHAPTER 7: ENVIRONMENT AND GENETIC IMPACT

1. Environmental hazards or risks coupled with genetic predisposition increase the likelihood of complex diseases. If exposed to adverse environments, it is not guaranteed complex disease may arise. It does, however, put certain populations at greater risk than others.
2. Autism, PD, and RSV
3. Understanding DNA expression as it relates to environmental stimuli can alert nurses to high-risk, vulnerable populations. Controlling and reasonably modifying environments can improve health outcomes if nurses include these concepts in their daily clinical application.

## CHAPTER 8: ETHICS AND GENETICS

1. B. Beneficence
2. C. Intentional selection of embryos for implantation that pass disabilities onto their children
3. A. A moral law that must be followed in all circumstances
4. B. The action must be in accord with the natural functioning of the universe.
5. D. Kant

## CHAPTER 9: GENETICS AND THE LAW

1. E. A and C only
2. C. Health insuers cannot discrimate against insurees on the basis of genetics
3. C. Employers may not unlawfully acquire, use, or disclose their employees genetic information
4. E. B and C only
5. D. All of the above

## CHAPTER 10: GENETIC SCREENING

1. Genetic screening is testing a population of asymptomatic individuals to identify those who have a pathogenic DNA variant(s) that puts them at increased risk to have a particular genetic or inherited disease, develop a disease, and/or transmit a disease to offspring.

2. Cascade screening would be discussed with the patient. It is important to notify her biologic relatives and offer them genetic counseling and testing for the *BRCA1* gene pathogenic DNA variant. There are medical interventions they can undergo if they test positive for the pathogenic DNA variant that will help to reduce their risk for getting breast, ovarian, and other cancers.
3. A screen negative result on NIPS indicates your baby is not at increased risk for Down syndrome, and two other chromosomal abnormalities, Trisomy 13 and 18 (and sex chromosomes if they were tested and included on the report). Keep in mind, the screen negative result does not mean your baby is free from these conditions; however, the risk is so low that no further follow-up is necessary. Moreover, the screening was only done for these conditions, so we do not know if your baby has increased risk for any other genetic or medical conditions. If a concern develops later in the pregnancy, further evaluation may be necessary.
4. Professional organizations provide recommendations for preconceptual carrier screening. Their health care provider will recommend carrier screening for cystic fibrosis and spinal muscular atrophy, and appropriate inherited conditions noted in their family history and specific ethnic group(s). Expanded carrier screening will also be recommended; however, the specific DNA variants associated with genetic conditions included on the panel depend on which guidelines their health care provider follows. Their health care provider may refer them to a professional genetic counselor. The couple should receive genetic counseling regarding general information on the conditions on the panel that are screened, risks and benefits of screening, the limitations of screening, and implications of possible results, including positive and negative results and potential impact on reproductive options. Screening is voluntary. Cost of screening may or may not be covered by insurance, so the couple needs to check with their insurer.
5. Newborn Screening. Each state manages their newborn screening program and determines the conditions screened. The RUSP serves as a guide with the recommended 35 disorders for which states screen. See Baby's First Test (n.d.) for a list of conditions screened and other information about newborn screening in their state.

## CHAPTER 13: PHARMACOGENOMICS

1. Pharmacogenetics focuses on the influence of single genes on drug response, and pharmacogenomics employs a broader view of the influence of an individual's entire genome on their drug response.

2. The cytochrome P 450 (CYP 450s) are a group of heme-conforming enzymes responsible for phase I and phase II metabolic reactions upon various drugs to activate or inactivate the drug response.
3. A pharmacogenomics test may be ordered to ascertain if the patient has a specific single-nucleotide polymorphism (SNP)/single-nucleotide variant (SNV) that would impact the metabolism of various drugs.

## CHAPTER 14: GENETIC TECHNOLOGY

1. The summation of DNA and cellular expression within a cell is referred to as the epigenome (Simmet et al., 2021).
2. Pluripotent cells are a subset of stem cells that have the potential to differentiate into almost any tissue or organ with exception of extraembryonic structures like the placenta and amnion.
3. DNA that is interrupted or broken is repaired by a process that is called nonhomologous end joining (NHEJ) or homologous recombination (HR) (Li et al., 2020).
4. Single-guide RNA (sgRNA) is an engineered tool utilized in the CRISPR-Cas9 system to accurately edit DNA. sgRNA consists of a sequence of nucleotides created in a lab. The sequence is palindromic to a gene of interest. When properly aligned, the CRISPR-Cas9 system will strike, creating double-strand breaks at this position. If the sgRNA is instructions for a working gene, function of the gene can be restored within the genome This process is called homology-directed repair (HDR). (Li et al., 2020).

## CHAPTER 15: GENOMICS IN HEALTHCARE

1. All of the above.
2. Integration of information on genomics, environment, personal and lifestyle factors, culture, and the environment to inform healthcare decision-making.
3. Enhanced education and workforce development and infrastructure and resources that support incorporation of genomics in practice.
4. Yes.

# Index

www.ingramcontent.com/pod-product-compliance
Ingram Content Group UK Ltd.
Pitfield, Milton Keynes, MK11 3LW, UK
UKHW021353110926
15107UKWH00004B/9

9 780826 184573